APPLIED NEUROPSYCHOLOGY

Editor-in-Chief
B. P. Uzzell, *Houston, Texas, USA*

Book & Test Review Editor
Nick A. DeFilippis, *Atlanta, Georgia, USA*

First published 2003 by Lawrence Erlbaum Associates, Inc.

This edition published 2016 by Routledge.
711 Third Avenue, New York, NY 10017
2 Park Square, Milton Park, Abingdon, Oxon OX14 4RN

Routledge is an imprint of the Taylor & Francis Group, an informa business.

ISBN 13: 978-0-8058-9615-2 (pbk)

Applied Neuropsychology is abstracted or indexed in *Index Medicus/MEDLINE; PsycINFO/Psychological Abstracts; EMBASE/Excerpta Medica; Cambridge Scientific Abstracts: Health & Safety Science; EBSCOhost Products; Risk Abstracts; Linguistics and Language Behavior Abstracts; ScienceDirect Navigator.* Microform copies of this journal are available through Bell & Howell Information and Learning, P.O. Box 1346, Ann Arbor, MI 48106–1346 USA. For more information, call 1-800-521-0600, x2888.

Applied Neuropsychology
2003, Vol. 10, No. 1, 1–3

INTRODUCTION

Sports-Related Concussions

Eric A. Zillmer

Department of Athletics, Drexel University, Philadelphia, Pennsylvania, USA

What role should the neuropsychologist have in the diagnosis, treatment, and management of sports-related concussions? This question is the focus of this special issue on sports-related concussions. I believe this to be a timely topic, as reports show mild traumatic brain injuries in multiple sports to be a consistently increasing trend over the past several years (e.g., Fall Sports Injury Research, 2002). Much attention has been given to the study of sports-related concussions, and great strides have been made in understanding this health concern, including the cultivation of neuropsychological assessment tools to diagnose concussions and the refinement of recovery curves after injury. Concussion injuries are now thought of as significant neuropsychological events with very real long-term consequences (Zillmer & Spiers, 2001). Nevertheless, many issues related to the diagnosis, assessment, and management of concussions are akin to putting a complex puzzle together:

- What is the effect of age and gender in concussions?
- What neuropsychological tests are best suited to assess concussions?
- What is the gold standard for grading concussions?
- What return-to-play guidelines are most practical?

I believe neuropsychologists play, and will continue to play, an important role in assembling this complex puzzle.

As the director of athletics of a Division 1 National Collegiate Athletic Association (NCAA) program, I am confronted on a daily basis with health issues of student-athletes. This is one reason why intercollegiate athletic programs have sports medicine facilities staffed by full-time, certified trainers. Our athletic trainers specialize in the treatment of sports-related injuries, attend practices, and travel with the team. Intercollegiate sports medicine centers are often supervised by consulting physicians who specialize in sports medicine. Sometimes there is a consulting neuropsychologist available, but many times there is not. When Julie, a 19-year-old forward on our women's soccer team, had a concussion as the result of a head-to-head collision with an opposing player, a cascade of neuropsychological, medical, personal, and competitive issues were brought to the forefront. The complex issues that confronted the trainer, team physician, and coach, as well as the player, her family, and her team, were related to how severe of an injury Julie had sustained, how much she had recovered, and when she should be cleared to play again. Orthopedic injuries to the knee or ankle seem to be better understood by the player, family, and coach, but it is quite puzzling to many who follow or participate in sports just how an athlete can be sidelined by a concussion. Given the complexity of the interplay between the often ambiguous and transient medical symptoms of the player and the competitive nature of sports, the neuropsychologist can offer a clearer focus on assessing and managing athletes with concussions.

If the college sports arena is complicated, the high-school athletic environment is even more daunting. In high school athletics, coaching duties as well as sports medicine care are often performed by part-time staffs, which are assigned to several teams. At the high-school level, concussions may go unnoticed or unmanaged. This is of concern because high-school students may be more at risk for concussions due to their age and their lower skill level in playing the sport.

Requests for reprints should be sent to Eric A. Zillmer, 3141 Chestnut Street, Department of Atheletics, Drexel University, Philadelphia, PA 19104, USA. E-mail: zillmer@drexel.edu

For some time now, neuropsychologists have played a significant role at the professional level in the assessment and management of concussions. For example, neuropsychologists have been instrumental in implementing concussion-testing programs for the National Hockey League (Lovell, Echemendia, & Burke, in press). For the average neuropsychologist, it may prove difficult to break into the ranks of professional athletics, although there are still new teams forming, such as indoor football. Moreover, professional athletics is not for everyone. The stakes can be very high because of the tremendous asset some athletes represent to the team.

The goal of this special issue is not to provide a comprehensive review of the remarkable progress that has been made over the last 15 years in the area of sports-related concussions. Many excellent reviews are available and the interested reader is referred to them (e.g., Echemendia & Julian, 2001; Guskiewicz, 2001). Rather, the goal of this special issue is to examine the most current issues facing us in this growing and dynamic field of neuropsychology. In the absence of any detectable abnormalities on traditional magnetic resonance imaging scans for cases with concussion (Bigler & Snyder, 1995), the objective nature of neuropsychological testing has become a reliable and valid approach to measuring cognitive impairment and symptom resolution for mild traumatic brain injury.

The first article in this special issue, by McKeever and Schatz, is dedicated to reviewing current issues in the neuropsychological assessment of concussions in sports-related injuries, including sideline assessment of concussions, serial postconcussion assessment, baseline testing, and computerized assessment.

Since Congress has passed Title IX in 1972 (i.e., legislation that prohibits educational institutions from practicing gender discrimination), the number of female varsity athletes in college has quadrupled. At Drexel University, for example, females make up 38% of the student body, but women participation on varsity sports teams is over 44%, earning Drexel Athletics a number one ranking in gender equity by *U.S. News & World Report* (Schneider, 2002). With this type of increased participation in contact sports, including ice hockey, lacrosse, soccer, and rugby, there has been a concomitant increase in the risk of sports-related concussions among female athletes. The contribution by Covassin, Swanik, and Sachs examines data, covering a period of 3 years, on over 6 million practice- and game-exposures among athletes participating in the NCAA Injury Surveillance System. Any neuropsychologist who wishes to work in the area of sports-related concussions must understand the epidemiology of the injuries they are assessing and how they differ by sport and gender.

Two contributions, by Zillmer and by Webbe and Ochs, examine the empirical role that neuropsychologists can have in the area of concussion research. These studies represent sports-related research that has immediate application for neuropsychologists in the field. Because many neuropsychologists have substantial knowledge in research design, I urge my colleagues to initiate or participate in the creation of data banks and multidisciplinary research projects as a means of studying concussions. Multidisciplinary research is also an excellent vehicle to initiate a dialogue among the different professions that provide clinical care and study concussions. For example, just this year my colleagues from two major universities and I have created the Philadelphia Sports Concussion Project to coordinate a central data bank for the participating five college athletic programs. Committee membership includes students, staff, and researchers from neuropsychology, athletic training, kinesiology, sports psychology, and sports medicine. Our monthly meetings have proven to be a terrific and stimulating vehicle for discussing relevant issues in the assessment and management of this complex injury.

Given that there are approximately 300,000 sports-related concussions reported each year (Thurman & Guerrero, 1999), computerized testing for the assessment of sports-related concussions may well be the wave of the future. It saves time, allows for team baseline testing, and can be easily incorporated into the sports medicine environment. The article on computer-based assessment of sports-related concussions by Schatz and Zillmer reviews the advantages and limitations of this approach.

The final article, by Echemendia and Cantu, discusses neuropsychology's role in return-to-play decisions following sports-related concussion. The article offers a model for such decisions and practical advice for neuropsychologists working in this multidisciplinary field.

Competitive sport participation has increased worldwide, and sports-related concussions represent a significant potential health concern to all of those who participate in contact sports. The role of the neuropsychologist in testing for concussions for purposes of diagnosis and symptom resolution is one that our profession should embrace. Moreover, for those neuropsychologists who love sports, it provides a unique opportunity to merge one's professional skills with one's affinity for sports. Most often, the role of the neuropsychologist in the area of sports-related concussions will be that of a consultant. Besides being an expert in the neuropsychological assessment of concussions, the neuropsychologist must understand the culture of the athletic arena and the various sports they may be asked to cover. I believe that the neuropsychologists' training and expertise uniquely prepares him or her to play an important and rewarding role in this growing field.

I thank all the authors and reviewers for their support of this project. Special appreciation goes to the editor-in-chief, Barbara Uzzell, who had the vision to include this emerging topic in the area of applied neuropsychology. I hope that this special issue will be of benefit to all neuropsychologists practicing in the field of sports-related concussions and serve as an inspiration for those who want to enter it.

References

Bigler, E. D., & Snyder, J. L. (1995). Neuropsychological outcome and quantitative neuroimaging in mild head injury. *Archives of Clinical Neuropsychology, 10,* 159–174.

Echemendia, R. J., & Julian, L. J. (2001). Mild traumatic brain injury in sports: Neuropsychology's contribution to a developing field. *Neuropsychology Review, 11,* 69–88.

Fall sports injury research indicates continued concern with concussions. (2002, April). *The NCAA News,* 10.

Guskiewicz, K. M. (Ed.). 2001. Concussion in athletes [Special issue]. *Journal of Athletic Training, 36*(3).

Lovell, M., Echemendia, R., & Burke, K. (in press). Neuropsychological assessment in professional hockey. In M. Lovell, R. Echemendia, J. Barth, & M. Collins (Eds.), *Sports neuropsychology.* Lisse, The Netherlands: Swets & Zeitlinger.

Schneider, J. (2002, March 18). America's best college sports programs: A guide to over 300 schools. *U.S. News & World Report,* 63–65.

Thurman, D., & Guerrero, J. (1999). Trends in hospitalization associated with traumatic brain injury. *Journal of the American Medical Association, 282,* 954–957.

Zillmer E. A., & Spiers, M. V. (2001). *Principles of neuropsychology.* Belmont, CA: Wadsworth.

Original submission May 1, 2002
Accepted August 9, 2002

Applied Neuropsychology
2003, Vol. 10, No. 1, 4–11

ARTICLES

Current Issues in the Identification, Assessment, and Management of Concussions in Sports-Related Injuries

Catherine K. McKeever

Department of Psychology, Drexel University, Philadelphia, Pennsylvania, USA

Philip Schatz

Department of Psychology, Saint Joseph's University, Philadelphia, Pennsylvania, USA

The recent literature has focused on the need for appropriate identification, assessment, and management of sports-related concussion. This article addresses current issues in the prevalence and assessment of sports-related concussion. Despite a paucity of research on female athletes and youth athletes, there is evidence that female athletes are at higher risk for injury than males and that concussions may affect children and young adolescents differently than older adolescents and adults. Sideline, baseline, and postconcussion assessments have become prevalent in documenting preinjury and postinjury performance, tracking recovery rates, and assisting return-to-play decisions. New computerized assessment procedures are growing in popularity and use. Future directions in the assessment and management of sports-related concussion include increased research on prevalence rates and effects of concussions for females and youth athletes, educating parents of youth athletes as well as family physicians on the importance of baseline and postconcussion cognitive assessments, and further validation of computerized assessment measures.

Key words: concussion, sports-related injury, mild traumatic brain injury, neuropsychological assessment, athletes, computerized assessment, baseline assessment, sideline assessment

Assessment of sports-related concussion has received considerable attention within the field of neuropsychology over the past decade. Specific research and applications have focused on a mechanism and pathophysiology of injury, the grading of concussions and recovery rates, return-to-play guidelines, and the development and validation of neuropsychological assessment measures. Important issues, such as the scarcity of research on the incidence of concussions in youth and female athletes, and the recent trend toward standardized and computerized assessment measures are, however, not as well represented in the current literature. It is the intention of this article to focus on neuropsychology's contributing role in the identification, assessment, and management of these emergent issues.

Prevalence of Sports-Related Concussions

Sports-related injuries represent approximately 20% of the estimated 1.54 million head injuries that occur yearly in the United States. Nine percent of all sports injuries are thought to be concussions (Erlanger, Kutner, Barth, & Barnes, 1999), and between 2% and 10% of all athletes are at risk for sustaining a concussion (Ruchinskas, Francis, & Barth, 1997). It is estimated that 10% of all college and 20% of all high

Requests for reprints should be sent to Philip Schatz, Department of Psychology, Saint Joseph's University, Philadelphia, PA 19131, USA. E-mail: pschatz@sju.edu school football injuries will be head injuries, which amounts to approximately 250,000 annually. Collins, Grindell, et al. (1999) found that 34% of 393 college football players had sustained at least one concussion and 20% reported a history of two or more concussions while on the team. During the 1997–1998 and 1998–1999 football seasons, 21% of football players were found to have had concussions, the majority of which were mild or Grade 1 according to the American Academy of Neurology (AAN) severity grading guidelines (Kelly & Rosenberg, 1997).

Although concussion in professional and college athletes is widely reported in the literature, concussion in high school athletes has only recently begun to receive similar attention. Powell and Barber-Foss (1999) estimated the number of concussions in high school varsity athletics to be 63,000. During a 3-year time span, 5.5% of all sports-related injuries reported among 235 high schools were concussions. Sports-related head injuries are most likely to occur among adolescents playing football (Baker & Patel, 2000). Powell and Barber-Foss (1999) found that 63.4% of sports-related injuries in high school football were concussions. Other activities in which youth athletes sustain sports-related concussions include wrestling, soccer, basketball, softball, baseball, field hockey, and volleyball.

Incidence of sports-related concussion appears to be increasing as a function of the number of the total sports activities, the number of previous sports years of the youth athlete, the recentness of the study, and the level of athletic participation (e.g., high school vs. college). Barth et al. (1989) reported that 10% of college football players in the Virginia football study sustained concussions each year, and 42% of their sample had sustained at least one previous concussion. Since then, incidence of previous concussion appears to have increased for collegiate athletes. Similarly, high school athletes appear to be sustaining concussions at a greater rate, as compared to collegiate athletes participating in the same sport. For example, concussion rates among college soccer players are estimated to be approximately 1 per 3,000 athletic exposures (AE; Green & Jordan, 1998). In contrast, concussion rates among high school soccer players have been reported to be higher at 1 per 2000 playing hours (Boden, Kirkendall, & Garrett, 1998). Between 7% and 11% of all sports-related injuries sustained by Canadian amateur hockey players aged 15 to 20 (over the 1998–1999 and 1999–2000 seasons) were concussions; 60% of these reported having sustained at least one concussion during either a game or practice (Goodman, Gaetz, & Meichenbaum, 2001). Moser and Schatz (2002) recently reported that 97% of athletes age 14 to 19 years, sampled from a boarding school with mandatory sports participation requirements and who had participated in numerous sports over a period of many years, had sustained at least one previous sports-related concussion.

Younger athletes appear to be at increased risk for concussions. Giza and Hovda (2001) discussed the potential vulnerability of youth athletes who sustain concussions during critical stages in brain development, especially during a time of increased plasticity. They hypothesize that concussions in the developing brain may ultimately impair this plasticity; however, it is not yet clear whether this impairment is permanent or temporal. It is possible that participants in the initial Virginia football study represented youth athletes from a different culture or with a different history of athletic participation. College athletes from the mid-1980s would have been participating in little league and club sports in the 1970s, whereas high school athletes in the late 1990s were participating in such sports activities in the late 1980s and early 1990s. Although there is no empirical data available on this specific variable, Moser and Schatz's (2002) sample was comprised of youth athletes with an average of 5 to 7 previous years of participation, as well as current participation in multiple sports. It is unlikely that athletes from the 1980s were being shuttled from soccer to lacrosse to baseball practice by era-equivalent "soccer moms." Thus, it appears that there may be a higher chance of sustaining concussive injuries when an athlete participates in more sports, has played for a higher number of years, and competes during high school years or earlier.

Additionally, the higher incidence of concussion rates in adolescents may simply be the result of younger, more susceptible brains. Although overall survival from severe head injury may be more likely in the pediatric population than in adults (Tepas, DiScala, Ramenofsky, & Barlow, 1990), traumatic brain injury in children and adolescents can lead to persistent cognitive dysfunction, even when no initial effects are observed (Giza & Hovda, 2001). Increased susceptibility to concussion in children and adolescents, as compared to adults, has been attributed to decreased myelination, a greater head-to-body ratio, and thinner cranial bones, all which provide less protection to the developing cortex.

The number of sports-related concussions appears to be increasing, and they are prevalent in all levels of sports participation. With the pervasive nature of sports-related concussion comes the need for appropriate identification by professionals, such as neuropsychologists, who are trained to investigate such injuries in a systematic and useful manner. Neuropsychologists have a knowledge base, which can contribute to an understanding of the susceptibility of sports-related concussion and different rates of recovery among disparate age groups. Integrating knowledge of the plasticity and repairing mechanisms of the brain, along with a comprehensive understanding of cognitive functions, neuropsychologists can provide unique insight to identifying and managing sports-related injuries in children, adolescents, young adults, and older adults.

Gender Differences

The National Athletic Trainers' Association study was the first major research effort delineating at-risk concussion differences between male and female athletes (Powell & Barber-Foss, 1999). In this study, female athletes were consistently found to be at higher risk for sustaining concussions than male athletes participating in the same high school sport: 1.14 concussions (per 100 player-seasons) in girls soccer versus .92 in boys soccer, 1.04 in girls basketball versus .75 in boys basketball, and .46 in girls softball versus .23 in boys baseball. These gender disparities represent approximate female-to-male concussion ratios of 5:4 for soccer, 4:3 for basketball, and 2:1 for softball and baseball. Similarly, Dick (1999) presented data from the National Collegiate Athletic Association (NCAA) Injury Surveillance System in which female athletes were at nearly twice the risk for concussion than male athletes playing soccer (.578 vs. .348 injuries per 1,000 AE) and lacrosse (.618 vs. .334 per 1,000 AE).

These trends do not appear to carry over to all sports or to athletes of all age ranges. Concussion rates in college soccer players (0.31 per 1,000 AE for male athletes and 0.33 per 1,000 AE for female athletes; Green & Jordan, 1998) and basketball players (36.8% of males, 31.3% of females; Echemendia, 1997) were found to be nearly identical for both genders. Barnes et al. (1998), however, observed that 78% of head injuries incurred by female athletes in Olympic soccer matches were the result of a collision with another player, as compared to 65% of head injuries for male athletes. Differences in brain chemistry and other as yet under-investigated neuroanatomical differences may account for this disparity; nevertheless, it is not yet clear why female athletes are at higher risk for sustaining concussions than male athletes.

Contrary to these findings, Boden et al. (1998) postulate that participants in boys soccer tend to represent a higher incidence of head injuries than girls soccer,

perhaps due to boys' greater willingness to engage in risk-taking behaviors. This trend toward increased risk-taking may explain why 89% of male versus 43% of female Olympic soccer players reported a prior history of concussion (Barnes et al. 1998).

Even if female athletes are sustaining concussions at the same rate as male athletes, there is a lack of data, research, and focus on female concussions. Although many research efforts focus on NCAA Division I football, a uniquely male sport, the overwhelming majority of studies representing sports such as soccer, rugby, basketball, and lacrosse are based primarily on male participants. An ideal manner by which to address this need can be met by neuropsychological research, which offers the unique opportunity to investigate the potentially different neuroanatomical and neurochemical elements that contribute to the distinct rates of sports-related concussions sustained by female athletes versus male athletes. Neuropsychological investigation into the possible disparities between female performance and male performance on neurocognitive tests can be used not only to detect impairment following concussion but also provide insight into the potentially higher risk for concussion in females (see also Covassin, Swanik, & Sachs, this issue).

Assessment of Concussion

More than a decade after the publication of the Virginia football study (Alves, Rimel, & Nelson, 1987; Barth, et al. 1989), researchers continue to refine assessment protocols and add to the current literature in the areas of neuropsychology, sports medicine, and athletic training. Recent publications focus on guidelines for immediate postconcussion sideline assessments (McCrea, 2001), implementation of testing programs (Randolph, 2001), the sensitivity and specificity of standardized measures (Barr & McCrea, 2001), and statistical methods for documenting postconcussion changes (Daniel et al. 1999; Hinton-Bayre, Geffen, Geffen, McFarland, & Friis, 1999). The literature is replete with comprehensive reviews of historical aspects of and emergent trends in the assessment of sports-related concussion (Bleiberg, Halpern, Reeves, & Daniel, 1998; Echemendia & Julian, 2001; Grindel, Lovell & Collins, 2001; Lovell & Collins, 1998; Ruchinskas et al., 1997). Current research trends reflect the importance of sideline assessments, the inclusion of baseline assessments in concussion management and assessment, and the introduction and utility of computerized assessment batteries.

Sideline assessment of concussion. The Standardized Assessment of Concussion (SAC) was developed in accordance with guidelines set forth by the AAN and in response to the recommendation for the development of a standardized tool with which concussion could be immediately evaluated on the sidelines (McCrea, Kelly, Kluge, Ackley, & Randolph, 1997). The SAC is comprised of four components: orientation, immediate memory, concentration, and delayed recall. Benefits include ease and brevity of administration and scoring and alternate forms for follow-up assessment and tracking recovery. Validation studies reveal the SAC to be accurate in classifying concussed athletes from nonconcussed controls with 95% sensitivity and 76% specificity (Barr & McCrea, 2001; McCrea, 2001).

More recently, Erlanger, Feldman, and Kutner (1999) developed the eSAC, which is essentially an electronic version of the SAC that can be used to administer sideline assessments using a Palm handheld or equivalent personal digital assistant. As with the original version of the SAC, alternate test forms are available to monitor postconcussion progress and recovery. The eSAC also stores information about athletes that may be useful to athletic trainers on the sideline, such as a roster of all athletes, their emergency contact numbers, and pertinent medical information.

Concussed athletes have displayed deficits in immediate memory and delayed recall, as well as significantly decreased performance on postconcussion test trials in comparison to individual baseline test performance on the SAC (McCrea et al., 1998). As such, McCrea (2001) recommended that the SAC not be used as a stand-alone tool and that optimal evaluation of sports-related concussion occurs with information from the SAC, additional comprehensive neuropsychological test measures, physical examinations, and the player's self-report of postconcussive symptoms. Further, Collins, Lovell, and McKeag (1999) stated that sideline assessments provide only gross indications of the injured athlete's cognitive abilities and deficits, and return-to-play decisions should not be determined based solely on these results.

Nevertheless, the usefulness of a sideline assessment tool, such as the SAC or the eSAC, to immediately and accurately detect mental status changes related to sports-related concussion will assist in the diagnosis and management of this complex injury. Further neuropsychological research into the identification of concussion utilizing such measures will lead to better delineation of the acute effects of sports-related concussive injuries.

Baseline and serial postconcussion assessment. Assessments used to document preconcussion and postconcussion performance tend to be more detailed and include more complex tasks than either sideline assessments or other screening measures that may take only 5 to 10 min to complete. Baseline assessments provide a vital experimental control for individual differences among players. Those individuals who, relative to other athletes, perform poorly on baseline measures cannot be classified as injured due to poor subsequent performances on the tests. Knowledge of an athlete's premorbid level of functioning is important (Bernhardt, 2000), especially when attempting to determine whether an impairment seen on postconcussion cognitive testing is due to the effects of a recent concussion compared to an individual's relative weakness in that cognitive domain.

Researchers have employed brief batteries of specific tests (Barth et al., 1989) as well as more comprehensive neuropsychological test batteries (Echemendia & Julian, 2001; Lovell & Collins, 1998) to assess sports-related concussive injuries. In contrast to brief test batteries or sideline assessments, more comprehensive neuropsychological test batteries are typically reserved for cases in which there is a question of permanent cognitive impairment, a history of multiple concussions, or when repetitive baseline tests may have confounded results due to practice effects (Randolph, 2001). Formal neuropsychological assessment tools have been shown to be both reliable and valid in the detection of concussion, and they have been used to provide specific scientific data to determine the presence of a concussion, document an injured athlete's fitness to return to play, track recovery curves, and protect against catastrophic injuries related to either multiple concussions or second-impact syndrome (Barth, Freeman, Broshek, & Varney, 2001).

Completion of baseline neuropsychological testing has been universally recommended for the purposes of comparison with postconcussion assessment data. The aforementioned Virginia football studies (Alves et al., 1987; Barth et al., 1989) were the first published studies to incorporate formal neuropsychological assessment measures in detecting residual effects of concussion in collegiate football players. In this study, serial assessment, for which the injured athlete was matched with an uninjured athlete to control for practice effects, occurred at 2 hr, 48 hr, 1 week, and 1 month postinjury to track recovery and to determine the concussed athlete's fitness to return to play. Serial assessments can demonstrate gradual improvement or deterioration in mental status over time, allow for better differentiation of cognitive deficits, and assist in treatment and management of concussions. This original pattern of serial assessment allowed for the determination of the time when an athlete's concussion symptoms were resolved, which was found to occur between 5 and 10 days postinjury. Since that time, various test measures and schedules for postconcussion serial assessments have been employed, each contributing differently to the understanding of the postconcussion recovery trajectory for various sports or preinjury conditions. Selected studies demonstrating various schedules of serial postconcussion assessment and test batteries are presented in Table 1. As can be seen from Table 1, there is little agreement regarding the schedule of serial testing to evaluate symptom resolution of concussed athletes, nor is there conformity on the neuropsychological procedures used to document the cognitive changes. Although the diversity of test measures and assessment schedules has provided an increased understanding of postconcussion recovery patterns, these between-study differences preclude collaborative data sharing or cross-comparisons at specific time intervals.

Preconcussion and postconcussion testing by neuropsychologists provides a comprehensive approach to identifying a concussion and documenting the effects on cognition. Most importantly, testing provides the opportunity to use objective data of symptom resolution in making return-to-play decisions (see also Echemendia & Cantu, this issue). Without the use of baseline and subsequent serial testing, there is no assurance that a concussed athlete is neuropsychologically fit to return to athletic participation where reaction time and decision-making capabilities are critical not only for skilled participation but also for protection against further injury.

Computerized assessment. Evaluations of entire athletic teams or programs have been identified as being both time- and labor-intensive, thus burdening financial resources and creating potential reluctance on the part of the school or facility (Maroon et al., 2000). Brief screening batteries, comprised of carefully selected measures may, in part, help lessen these burdens (Lovell & Collins, 1998). However, any repetitive or serial assessment will expose athletes to test measures over multiple sessions, thereby creating unwanted and often confounding practice effects. Such practice effects can introduce error into assessment data, obscure the effects of concussion, and, ultimately, compromise the reliability of the assessment (Hinton-Bayre et al., 1999). Additionally, practice effects have been shown to vary from test to test and across serial assessment intervals (Heaton et al., 2001), further complicating and compromising the reliability and interpretation of postconcussion test data.

Cerebral concussions have been shown to cause subtle deficits in speed and quality of information processing (Moser & Schatz, 2002). Tests that measure attention, concentration, reaction time, psychomotor coding, and working memory are most commonly utilized in baseline and postconcussion evaluations (Barth et al., 1989; Collins, Lovell, et al., 1999; Echemendia & Julian, 2001; Lovell & Collins, 1998). Concussed individuals have been shown to differ significantly from otherwise healthy controls on tests of reaction time by margins of 110 ms or less (Bleiberg et al., 1998), and such measurement accuracy cannot be achieved with the traditional means of examiners using stopwatches.

A fully computerized battery may be the best approach to assessing sports-related concussions for several reasons (Randolph, 2001). First, the comprehensive battery can offer an objective approach to administration and scoring of test protocols. Second, time and cost constraints and the availability of personnel can be practically accommodated. Third, if a player moves from one team to another, as is often the case in professional sports, baseline data and any subsequent testing trials can easily be transferred from one database to another. Research efforts have focused on computerizing specific tests for the purpose of test validation (Hatfield, Laforce, Lapland, & Barite, 2001) or for use in assessment of sports-related concussion (Schatz & MacNamara, 2001). To date, however, only three computerized test batteries have been developed: the Immediate Measurement of Performance and Cognitive Testing (Lovell, Collins, Podell, Powell, & Maroon, 2000), the Concussion Resolution Index (Erlanger, Feldman, et al., 1999), and CogSport (CogState, 1999). Each of these batteries has been used effectively in the assessment of sports-related concussion (see also Schatz & Zillmer, this issue).

In sum, neuropsychologists can utilize computerized batteries in a time- and cost-efficient manner to effectively identify the presence of even the mildest of concussive injuries. Further, the results of such assessments can provide a sensitive vehicle by which to track recovery curves that can lead to comprehensive and realistic recommendations regarding an athlete's return to play.

Future Directions

As awareness of sports-related concussions is increasing, this issue has the potential to become a public health concern. There have been a number of studies examining the effects of concussion on both college and professional athletes, yet few studies incorporate

Table 1. *Comparison of Postconcussion Assessment Schedules*

Study	Schedule of Serial Postconcussion Assessments							Measures Used
	Hours		Days					
	1–2	24–48	3	5	7	10	30	
NCAA–Multiple sports (Echemendia et al., 2001)	2	24			7		30	PC, HVLT[a], SDMT, Stroop Test, Trails[b], VIGIL/W[c], Digit Span, PSU, COWAT
NCAA–Football (Collins et al., 1999)	1		3	5	7			HVLT[a], Trails[b], Digit Span, SDMT, COWAT, Pegboard[d]
NCAA–Football (Barth et al., 1989)		24		5		10		SDMT, Trails[b], PASAT
Prof. Hockey Players (Echemendia, 2001)		24		5[e]	7[e]			PC, HVLT[a], SDMT, Trails[f], PSU, COWAT, BVMT–R
Prof. Football Players (Lovell & Collins, 1998)		24		5				HVLT[a], SDMT, Trails[b], Digit Span, COWAT, Pegboard[d]
Prof. Rugby Players (McCrory et al., 1997)	1			5				SDMT, Choice RT[g], Memory[h], Orientation[h]
Prof. Rugby Players (Hinton-Bayre et al., 1999)			3[i]		7[i]		35[i]	SDMT, Digit Symbol[j], Speed of Comprehension[h]

Note: PC = Postconcussion Checklist; SDMT = Symbol Digit Modalities Test; PSU = Penn State University Cancellation Task; COWAT = Controlled Oral Word Association Test; PASAT = Paced Auditory Serial Addition Test; BVMT–R = Brief Visuospatial Motor Test–Revised. [a]Postconcussion Checklist. [b]Trail Making Test A & B. [c]Continuous Performance Task. [d]Grooved Pegboard Test. [e]Athletes tested 5 to 7 days postconcussion. [f]Color Trail Making Test. [g]Symbol Digit Modalities Test (with incidental memory testing). [h]Unspecified. [i]Athletes tested 1 to 3 days, 1 to 2 weeks, 3 to 5 weeks postconcussion. [j]Digit Symbol subtest of the Wechsler Adult Intelligence Scale–Revised.

high school athletes, and even fewer address female athletes. More research is needed to investigate the high prevalence of concussion and its potentially detrimental effects in youth athletes, a population engaging in more and more athletic activities at increasingly younger ages. Investigations examining the neuroanatomical differences and mechanisms of injury in child and adolescent athletes could also provide important information to physicians, athletic trainers, neuropsychologists, and parents. Such research may yield needed age-appropriate protective equipment, concussion-grading scales, return to play guidelines, and rules changes, such as those that have been introduced in the National Football League in the recent past.

Although neuropsychologists and athletic trainers appear to have an understanding of the potentially dangerous impact of concussions, there needs to be more widespread understanding of and support for these issues. Family physicians and pediatricians may or may not already be aware of the potential physical, emotional, and cognitive sequelae of concussion in athletes. These physicians can serve to educate parents about the risks involved in athletic activity and the need to seek professional services when sports-related injuries occur, especially when youth athletes are participating in athletic programs not mediated by sports-concussion management programs. Practicing neuropsychologists should recognize that parents and coaches are potentially the best resource for knowledge of the premorbid functions of the child athlete and in recognizing postinjury changes. To this end, parents are best suited to observe subsequent changes in their child off the field and thus seek professional help. Similarly, the education of coaches on the effects of concussion, and the importance of cognitive assessment after injury is essential. Together, physicians, parents, and coaches can help fulfill some of the roles now standard in many collegiate concussion management programs.

Assessment of neuropsychological sequelae following sports-related concussion and the recognition and management of symptoms are key to understanding the short- and long-term effects of concussion. Formal concussion management programs should be in place for every professional, semi-professional, college, high school, club team, little league, and youth sports program. Such programs are needed to identify physical and cognitive symptoms, to appropriately determine the need for more comprehensive neuropsychological assessment, to assist in determining fitness for returning to play, and to protect athletes against further concussion and second impact syndrome. Specifically, baseline, sideline, and serial assessment following

concussion can allow athletic programs to determine the severity of injury and safely return an athlete to play by formally tracking recovery rates.

Despite the considerable research on the cognitive effects of concussion, there is no common postconcussion assessment protocol currently in use. A core battery of tests that is both reliable and valid in identifying concussion, grading concussions more carefully, and tracking recovery rates more precisely is needed in the research investigating the appropriate assessment of concussion. Further, such research should collect data at common postconcussion time frames to allow for cross-sample comparisons and collaborative data sharing. Recently developed computerized assessment tools appear to provide significant gains, with respect to both cost and time efficiency, while providing useful and unique response-time data and test-retest reliability not available using traditional measures. The initial validation research regarding the psychometrics of these computerized measures is promising, and continued validation should result in widespread adoption of computerized concussion management programs at all levels.

In conclusion, we make the following recommendations. Increase research on sports-related concussion in youth athletes at the pee-wee, little league, club sport, grade school, junior high, and high school level. Increase research on sports-related concussion in female athletes competing at all age levels and in all sports categories. Establish universal protocols utilizing common baseline, sideline, and serial postconcussion measures and assessment schedules. Implement comprehensive concussion management programs involving players, coaches, trainers, athletic directors, and team physicians. And involve parents and pediatricians in concussion education programs promoting mandatory baseline assessments for all youth athletes who are at risk.

References

Alves, W. M., Rimel, R. W., & Nelson, W. E. (1987). University of Virginia prospective study of football-induced minor head injury: Status report. *Clinical Sports Medicine, 6,* 211–218.

Baker, R. J., & Patel, D. R. (2000). Sports related mild traumatic brain injury in adolescents. *Indian Journal of Pediatrics, 67,* 317–321.

Barnes, B. C., Cooper, L., Kirkendall, D. T., McDermott, T. P., Jordan, B. D., & Garrett, W. E., Jr. (1998). Concussion history in elite male and female soccer players. *American Journal of Sports Medicine, 26,* 433–438.

Barr, W. B., & McCrea, M. (2001). Sensitivity and specificity of standardized neurocognitive testing immediately following sports concussion. *Journal of the International Neuropsychological Society, 7,* 693–702.

Barth, J. T., Alves, W. M., Ryan, T. V., Macciocchi, S. N., Rimel, R. W., Jane, J. A., et al. (1989). Head injury in sports: Neuropsychological sequelae and recovery of function. In H. S. Levin, H. M. Eisenberg, & A. L. Benton (Eds.), *Mild head injury*. New York: Oxford Press.

Barth, J. T., Freeman, J. R., Broshek, D. K., & Varney, R. N. (2001). Acceleration-deceleration sport-related concussion: The gravity of it all. *Journal of Athletic Training, 36*, 253–256.

Bernhardt, D. T. (2000). Football: A case based approach to mild traumatic brain injury. *Pediatric Annals, 29*, 172–176.

Bleiberg, J., Halpern, E. L., Reeves, D., & Daniel, J. (1998). Future directions for the assessment of sports concussion. *Journal of Head Trauma Rehabilitation, 13*, 331–337.

Boden, B. P., Kirkendall, D. T., & Garrett, W. E. J. (1998). Concussion incidence in elite college soccer players. *American Journal of Sports Medicine, 26*(2), 238–241.

CogState, Ltd. (1999). CogSport [Computer software]. Parkville, Victoria, Australia: Author.

Collins, M. W., Grindel, S. H., Lovell, M. R., Dede, D. E., Moser, D. J., Phalin, B. R., et al. (1999). Relationship between concussion and neuropsychological performance in college football players. *Journal of the American Medical Association, 282*, 964–970.

Collins, M. W., Lovell, M. R., & McKeag, D. B. (1999). Current issues in managing sports-related concussion. *Journal of the American Medical Association, 282*, 2283–2285.

Daniel, J. C., Olesniewicz, M. H., Reeves, D. L., Tam, D., Bleiberg, J., Thatcher, R., et al. (1999). Repeated measures of cognitive processing efficiency in adolescent athletes: Implications for monitoring recovery from concussion. *Neuropsychiatry, Neuropsychology, and Behavioral Neurology, 12*, 167–169.

Dick, R. W. (1999). *NCAA Injury Surveillance System: 1984–91*. Overland Park, KS: National Collegiate Athletics Association.

Echemendia, R. J. (1997, November). *Neuropsychological assessment of college athletes: The Penn State Concussion Program*. Paper presented at the meeting of the National Academy of Neuropsychology, Las Vegas, NV.

Echemendia, R. J., & Julian, L. J. (2001). Mild traumatic brain injury in sports: Neuropsychology's contribution to a developing field. *Neuropsychological Review, 11*, 69–88.

Erlanger, D. M., Feldman, D. J., & Kutner, K. (1999). *Concussion resolution index*. New York: HeadMinder, Inc.

Erlanger, D. M., Kutner, K., Barth, J., & Barnes, R. (1999). The neuropsychology of sports-related head injury: From dementia pugilistica to post-concussion syndrome. *The Clinical Neuropsychologist, 13*, 193–210.

Giza, C. C., & Hovda, D. A. (2001). The neurometabolic cascade of concussion. *Journal of Athletic Training, 36*, 228–235.

Goodman, D., Gaetz, M., & Meichenbaum, D. (2001). Concussion in hockey: There is cause for concern. *Medicine, Science, Sports Exercise, 33*, 2004–2009.

Green, G.A., & Jordan, S.E. (1998). Are brain injuries a significant problem in soccer? [Abstract]. *Clinics in Sports Medicine, 17*, 795–809.

Grindel, S. H., Lovell, M. R., & Collins, M. W. (2001). The assessment of sport-related concussion: The evidence behind neuropsychological testing and management. *Clinical Journal of Sports Medicine, 11*, 134–143.

Hatfield, L., Laforce, R., Jr., Lapland, L., & Barite, P. (2001). Validity and reliability of a computerized version of the Trail-Making Test in young and older participants. *Archives of Clinical Neuropsychology, 16*, 828.

Heaton, R. K., Timken, N., Daiken, S., Available, N., Taylor, M. J., Marquette, T. D., et al. (2001). Detecting change: A comparison of three neuropsychological methods, using normal and clinical samples. *Archives of Clinical Neuropsychology, 16*, 75–91.

Hinton-Bayre, A. D, Geffen, G. M, Geffen, L. B, McFarland, K. A., & Friis, P. (1999). Concussion in contact sports: Reliable change indices of impairment and recovery. *Journal of Clinical Experimental Neuropsychology, 21*, 70–86.

Kelly, J. P., & Rosenberg, J. H. (1997). Diagnosis and management of concussion in sports. *Neurology, 48*, 575–580.

Lovell, M. R., & Collins, M. W. (1998). Neuropsychological assessment of the college football player. *Journal of Head Trauma Rehabilitation, 13*(2), 9–26.

Lovell, M. R., Collins, M. W., Podell, K., Powell, J., & Maroon, J. (2000). *Immediate post-concussion assessment and cognitive testing* (ImPACT). Pittsburgh, PA: NeuroHealth Systems, LLC.

Maroon, J. C., Lovell, M. R., Norwig, J., Podell, K., Powell, J. W., & Hartl, R. (2000). Cerebral concussion in athletes: Evaluation and neuropsychological testing. *Neurosurgery, 47*, 659–669.

McCrea, M. (2001). Standardized mental status testing on the sideline after sports-related concussion. *Journal of Athletic Training, 36*, 274–279.

McCrea, M., Kelly, J. P., Kluge, J., Ackley, B., & Randolph, C. (1997). Standardized assessment of concussion in football players. *Neurology, 48*, 586–588.

McCrea, M., Kelly, J. P., Randolph, C., Kluge, J., Bartolic, E., Finn, G., et al. (1998). Standardized assessment of concussion (SAC): On-site mental status evaluation of the athlete. *Journal of Head Trauma Rehabilitation, 13*, 27–35.

Moser, R. S., & Schatz, P. (2002). Enduring effects of concussion in youth athletes. *Archives of Clinical Neuropsychology, 17*, 81–90.

Powell, J. W., & Barber-Foss, K. D. (1999). Traumatic brain injury in high school athletes. *Journal of the American Medical Association, 282*, 958–963.

Randolph, C. (2001). Implementation of neuropsychological testing models for the high school, collegiate, and professional sport settings. *Journal of Athletic Training, 36*, 288–296.

Ruchinskas, R., Francis, J., & Barth, J. T. (1997). Mild head injury in sports. *Applied Neuropsychology, 4*, 43–49.

Schatz, P., & MacNamara, K. A. (2001). Enduring effects of previous concussion in college freshmen and sophomores. *Archives of Clinical Neuropsychology, 16*, 746.

Tepas, J. J., DiScala, C., Ramenofsky, M. L., & Barlow, B. (1990). Mortality and head injury: The pediatric perspective. *Journal of Pediatric Surgery, 25*, 92–96.

Original submission May 1, 2002
Accepted August 9, 2002

Applied Neuropsychology
2003, Vol. 10, No. 1, 12–22

Epidemiological Considerations of Concussions Among Intercollegiate Athletes

Tracey Covassin, C. Buz Swanik, and Michael L. Sachs

Department of Kinesiology, Temple University, Philadelphia, Pennsylvania, USA

The purpose of this study was to examine epidemiological trends of concussions among 15 different intercollegiate sports during the 1997–1998, 1998–1999, and 1999–2000 seasons. Data were collected using the National Collegiate Athletic Association (NCAA) Injury Surveillance System (ISS). For the 15 sports studied during the 3 academic years, the NCAA ISS documented 3,535 team-seasons, 40,547 reportable injuries, 5,566,924 practice athlete exposures (AEs), and 1,090,298 game AEs. Concussions accounted for 6.2% of all reported injuries during this 3-year study. Of all the reported injuries, women lacrosse players (13.9%) reported the highest percentage of suffering a concussion during a game followed by women's soccer (11.4%), men's ice hockey (10.3%), men's lacrosse (10.1%), football (8.8%), women's basketball, (8.5%), field hockey (7.2%), men's soccer (7.0%), wrestling (6.6%), men's basketball (5.0%), baseball (4.2%), and women's volleyball (4.1%). Female athletes from all 7 sports were found to be at a lower risk for suffering concussions during practice sessions than the 8 male sports. However, female athletes were found to be at a greater risk for suffering concussions during games compared to male athletes. Injury trends over the 3-year period indicate concussions continue to be on the rise for athletes participating in collegiate football, men's soccer, and women's and men's basketball.

Key Words: concussions, intercollegiate sports, male sports, female sports, National Collegiate Athletic Association, Injury Surveillance System, injury, athlete exposure, injury rate, incidence density ratio

In recent years there has been increasing interest in the effects and evaluation of concussions in sports. There are approximately 300,000 sport-related concussions reported each year (Thurman & Guerrero, 1999). Most sports, especially contact sports, have an inherent risk of injury to the brain. Although many concussions are considered minor, the cumulative effects of repeated concussions can have long-term consequences (Evans, 1994; Kelly, 1995). Furthermore, athletic trainers and team physicians have difficulty detecting and fully characterizing sport concussions on routine clinical examinations because the athletes' motivation to participate in athletics may cause them to minimize their symptoms so they can continue to participate (Evans, 1994; Kelly, 1995).

Since injury trends in concussions are important for the health and welfare of athletes and their treatment, there is a need to determine which athletes have a more inherent risk of suffering a concussion. Moreover, there is a need to determine if athletes have an increased risk of suffering a concussion during practice sessions or games. Determination of concussion risk is also important for future advances by the National Collegiate Athletic Association (NCAA) Committee on Competitive Safeguards and Medical Aspects of Sports so they can make changes as needed. However, it is difficult to determine the true risk of concussions and the number of concussions in athletes, which may potentially be related to how the profession defines concussions. The sports medicine community does not know for certain how concussions resolve or the wide nature of individual symptoms that are encountered in concussed athletes. Neuropsychologists are in a unique position to assist in the assessment, diagnosis, and management of sports-related concussions. It is impor-

Requests for reprints should be sent to C. Buz Swanik, Department of Kinesiology, Temple University, Pearson Hall #127, Philadelphia, PA 19122, USA.

tant for neuropsychologists practicing in this area to understand the epidemiological nuances among the different sports and trends over time. As neuropsychologists become increasingly informed about the complex culture of intercollegiate sports and specific base rates of concussion, the more effective they will be in becoming an important resource in this field.

Essentially, there is no universal agreement on the definition of concussion. The historical definition refers to its Latin origin, *concutere,* meaning "agitation or shaking" of the brain (Maroon et al., 2000). The American Medical Association and the Committee of Head Injury Nomenclature of the Congress of Neurological Surgeons (1966) defined *concussion* as a clinical syndrome characterized by the immediate and transient posttraumatic impairment of neurological function (such as alteration of consciousness, disturbance of vision and equilibrium), due to brainstem involvement. The Quality Standards Subcommittee of the American Academy of Neurology (AAN; 1997) described cerebral concussions as an altered mental state that may or may not include loss of consciousness. This committee agreed that the most prominent symptoms of concussions are amnesia and confusion (see also Echemendia & Cantu, this issue).

Research on three sports, including football, ice hockey, and soccer, is summarized in this article. These three sports represent different areas on which research attention has focused and thus a review of previous epidemiological data is offered here.

Concussions in Football Players

Until the 1980s, there was very little research being conducted on concussions. Gerberich, Priest, Boen, Straub, and Maxwell (1983) reported one of the first studies regarding incidence and severity of concussions in high school players. The researchers surveyed 103 secondary football teams in Minnesota during the 1977 football season. The authors concluded concussions accounted for 24% of all football injuries. However, this study was conducted 3 years prior to implementation of the rule mandating that all football helmets be required to meet approval by the National Operating Committee for Safety in Athletic Equipment. As a result of the helmet rule, concussion rates have dropped considerably, to approximately 5% (Barth et al., 1989; McCrea, Kelly, Kluge, Ackley, & Randolph, 1997; McCrea et al., 1998). Several other researchers have studied concussions in high school and college football players. Buckley (1988) examined 35,879 college football players between the 1975 to 1982 seasons. The researcher concluded that 5.3% of football players sustained a minor concussion with less than 7 days lost from participation. McCrea et al. (1997) examined 141 Iowa high school football players during the 1995 football season. Six athletes suffered a Grade 2 concussion, which accounted for 4.3% of all football injuries.

Due to a high percentage of football players suffering concussions, the Quality Standards Committee of the AAN recommended the development of the Standardized Assessment of Concussions (SAC). The SAC provides immediate sideline neurocognitive impairment assessment of athletes who have just sustained a concussion (McCrea et al., 1998). The SAC was developed to aid in sideline evaluation for certified athletic trainers and physicians and is similar to a mental status evaluation; however, it does not replace a comprehensive neuropsychological test battery. McCrea et al. (1998) administered the SAC to 568 nonconcussed high school and college football players prior to the start of the season. Thirty-three athletes (5.8%) suffered a concussion during the season. They scored significantly below their own preinjury baseline score on the SAC. Similar results were reported by Barth et al. (1989), who indicated that 7.7% of all football players sustained a mild head injury during the season.

Very few studies have been published on professional football players. Delaney, Lacroix, Leclerc, and Johnson (2000) investigated the incidence and characteristics of concussions in professional football players in the Canadian Football League (CFL). All players completed a questionnaire about concussions they sustained during the 1997 CFL season. Players self-reported their signs and symptoms and the duration they were unable to play football. Results indicated that 8.4% recognized they had sustained a concussion during the season. However, 44.8% of players reported signs and symptoms of sustaining a concussion. The most common clinical symptoms of concussion were confusion, followed by headache, dizziness, and blurred vision. Results revealed that 69.6% of football players who experienced signs and symptoms of concussion reported more than one episode during the 1997 season.

If an athlete is experiencing postconcussion symptoms and returns to play prematurely, this may lead to catastrophic consequences (Cantu, 1996; Fekete, 1968; Kelly et al., 1991; McCrory & Berkovic, 1998; Saunders & Harbaugh, 1984). Second-impact syndrome occurs when an athlete sustains a second head injury while still recovering from the first head injury

(Cantu & Voy, 1995). Therefore, better tracking of concussions using neuropsychological procedures may help minimize the risk of second-impact syndrome and potential neuropsychological impairments.

Concussions in Ice Hockey Players

Ice hockey has recently had several prominent professional hockey players who were diagnosed with concussions or forced to retire due to numerous concussions. As a result, the National Hockey League (NHL) formed a committee to examine this increased incidence of concussions in hockey players. Tegner and Lorentzon (1996) examined the frequency of concussions among Swedish elite hockey players. The participants of the study represented 12 teams, with 628 games played and a total of 7,536 player-game-hours. Doctors diagnosed 52 concussions during the four ice hockey seasons (5%). The authors concluded that around 20% of all elite ice hockey players will sustain at least one concussion during their entire hockey career. Lorentzon, Wedren, and Pietila (1988) reported Swedish elite hockey players had a 5.3% risk of sustaining a concussion during a hockey season.

Concussions in Soccer Players

Several researchers have shown interest with regards to the prevalence and incidence of concussions among soccer players. Concussions have been reported to constitute 2% to 22% of all soccer injuries (Barnes et al., 1998; Boden, Kirkendall, & Garrett, 1998; Bruce, Schut, & Sutton, 1982; see also Webbe & Ochs, this issue). Boden et al. (1998) examined the mechanism and incidence of concussions in male and female varsity soccer players participating in the Atlantic Coast Conference. Results indicated that the concussion incidence for men was 0.6 per 1,000 athlete exposures (AEs) and 0.4 per 1,000 AEs for women over the two seasons studied. This supports Barnes et al.'s (1998) research, which concluded that men have a higher incidence of concussions than women and concussions are becoming more common than previously anticipated.

No studies to date have examined epidemiological injury trends over time on collegiate athletes who sustain a concussion. Therefore, the purpose of this study was to examine the incidence and prevalence of concussions among 15 different intercollegiate sports during the 1997–1998 to 1999–2000 seasons. A secondary goal of this study was to determine which sports are associated with a greater risk of suffering a concussion during games versus practice sessions.

Methods

Data were collected using the NCAA Injury Surveillance System (ISS) from 3,535 team-seasons. Certified athletic trainers from participating NCAA institutions recorded injury and AE data from the first day of preseason practice to the final postseason game. Data collected from each sports season (fall, winter, spring) were then summarized and reviewed by the NCAA Committee on Competitive Safeguards and Medical Aspects of Sports. The NCAA ISS was developed in 1982 to provide reliable and current data on injuries sustained by intercollegiate athletes (NCAA, 1997). During the 1982–1983 academic year, injury data were collected on football players only. By the 1999–2000 academic year, the NCAA ISS had expanded to 15 sports, including 5 fall sports (field hockey, football, men's soccer, women's soccer, and women's volleyball), 6 winter sports (men's basketball, women's basketball, men's gymnastics, women's gymnastics, men's ice hockey, and men's wrestling), and 5 spring sports (baseball, men's lacrosse, women's lacrosse, spring football, and softball).

Sampling

Participation in the NCAA ISS system was voluntary. Selection to participate in the ISS was random, but there is a minimum of 10% representation from each region (East, South, Midwest, and West) and NCAA division (I, II, and III). Therefore, NCAA ISS collected a random sample that is representative of a true cross section of NCAA institutions.

Terminology

The following terminology is used in this article:

- *National Collegiate Athletic Association (NCAA).* The NCAA acts as a governing body to establish rules and regulations in United States collegiate sports to provide for safer and fairer sports participation.
- *Injury Surveillance System (ISS).* The ISS collects yearly injury data from a representative sample of NCAA institutions.

- *Injury.* The ISS defined a reportable injury as one that occurs as a result of participation in an organized intercollegiate practice or game, requires medical attention by a team athletic trainer or physician, and results in restriction of the student-athlete's participation for one or more days beyond the day of injury.
- *Athlete Exposure (AE).* An AE is defined by the NCAA ISS as an athlete participating in one practice or game where she or he is exposed to the possibility of athletic injury. Certified athletic trainers submit a weekly exposure form, summarizing the number of practices and games. For example, four practices, each involving 15 participants, and two games involving 9 participants, would result in 60 practice AEs, 18 game AEs, and 78 total AEs for that week.
- *Injury Rate.* The NCAA ISS defines an injury rate as the ratio of the number of injuries in a sport to the number of athletes exposed to the same sport. Injury-rate values are expressed as injuries per 1,000 AEs.
- *Incidence Density Ratio (IDR).* The IDR is an estimate of the relative risk based on injury rates per 1,000 AEs. The IDR is a ratio comparing games to practice injury rates of athletes sustaining a concussion. It is calculated by dividing the injury rate of games by the injury rate of practice sessions. The IDR provides an indication of where risk is concentrated, either practices or games.

Statistical Analyses

Statistical analyses included chi-squares, the IDR, and the percentages of injuries that were classified as a concussion. Iteration proportion fitting chi-squares were conducted to create theoretical expected values. Chi-squares were performed to analyze differences between years, practice versus games, and among sports. The 95% confidence intervals were calculated according to the methods of Miettinen (1973). The Statistical Package for the Social Sciences, version 10.1, was used for all statistical analyses. The statistical significance level was set at $p < .01$.

Results

For the 15 sports studied during the 3 academic years, the NCAA ISS documented 3,535 team-seasons, 40,547 reportable injuries, 5,566,924 practice AEs, and 1,090,298 game AEs. Overall, 6.2% of all injuries suffered by both men and women were concussions. Of the reported injuries, 1,224 (1,224/24,480 = 5.0%) concussions were sustained during practice and 1,278 (1,278/15,975 = 8.0%) were sustained during games. Female athletes sustained 191 (191/5,788 = 3.3%) concussions during practices and 331 (331/3,719 = 8.9%) concussions during games. Male athletes sustained 1,033 (1,033/18,782 = 5.5%) concussions during practices and 947 (947/12,299 = 7.7%) concussions during games. Data for practice and game concussions are shown in Tables 1 through 4.

Chi-square analysis revealed statistical significance between male games and male practice session for football ($\chi^2 = 734.9$), soccer ($\chi^2 = 323.1$), ice hockey ($\chi^2 = 141.7$), lacrosse ($\chi^2 = 82.3$), wrestling ($\chi^2 = 63.9$), baseball ($\chi^2 = 50.2$), and basketball ($\chi^2 = 24.7$; see Table 1). Chi-square analyses revealed statistical significance between female games and female practices for soccer ($\chi^2 = 478.83$), basketball ($\chi^2 = 45.33$), lacrosse ($\chi^2 = 23.74$), and field hockey ($\chi^2 = 8.11$; see Table 3). Results revealed the highest IDR for male games to practices were the 1999–2000 soccer (39.00), 1998–1999 lacrosse (22.57), 1997–1998 wrestling (18.10), and the 1997–1998 ice hockey (17.35) seasons (see Table 1). The highest IDR for female games to practices were the 1998–1999 (18.64), 1999–2000 (17.00), and 1997–1998 (14.57) soccer seasons and the 1998–1999 field hockey (10.5) season (see Table 3). Of all the reported male game injuries, the 1999–2000 lacrosse (11.9%) players suffered the highest percentage of concussions, followed by the 1999–2000 ice hockey (11.6%), 1997–1998 wrestling (10.9%), and 1997–1998 ice hockey (10.2%) seasons (see Table 1). Of all the reported male practice injuries, the 1997–1998 ice hockey (7.9%) players reported the highest percentage of concussions, followed by the 1998–1999 spring football (7.4%), 1999–2000 football (7.2%), and 1998–1999 football (6.7%), and 1999–2000 spring football (6.7%; see Table 2). The highest percentage of concussions reported for female games were the 1997–1998 lacrosse (16%), 1998–1999 lacrosse (13.5%), 1999–2000 lacrosse (12.1%), and 1999–2000 soccer seasons (12.1%; see Table 3). The highest percentage of concussions reported for female practice sessions were 1997–1998 lacrosse (8.9%), 1997–1998 field hockey (5.4%), 1999–2000 basketball (5.1%), and 1999–2000 softball (4.9%; see Table 4).

Table 1. *Male Game Concussions*

Sport	Year	Total Games	Total Number of Injuries	Total Concussions	Concussion Injury Rates[a]	Percentage of Concussions[b]	IDR[c]	Chi-Square[d]
Hockey	97–98	19,005	362	37	2.95	10.2%	17.35	141.7*
	98–99	14,080	239	20	1.42	8.4%	14.2	
	99–00	21,462	362	42	1.96	11.6%	15.08	
Lacrosse	97–98	13,486	213	19	1.41	8.9%	10.07	82.3*
	98–99	9,514	156	15	1.58	9.6%	22.57	
	99–00	12,177	143	17	1.39	11.9%	7.32	
Football	97–98	52,317	1,795	121*	2.32	6.7%	10.9	734.9*
	98–99	52,505	1,776	137*	2.61	7.7%	3.0	
	99–00	67,393	3,022	280*	4.15	9.3%	5.9	
Wrestling	97–98	10,422	311	34*	3.26	10.9%	18.1	63.9*
	98–98	5,169	132	4*	0.77	3.0%	2.2	
	99–00	9,807	305	18	1.84	5.9%	5.9	
Soccer	97–98	30,966	549	34	1.10	6.2%	13.75	323.1*
	98–99	19,142	376	27	1.41	7.2%	12.82	
	99–00	25,636	529	40	1.56	7.6%	39.00	
Basketball	97–98	27,706	220	8	0.29	3.6%	2.07	24.7*
	98–99	39,367	402	21	0.26	5.2%	1.37	
	99–00	32,836	327	20	0.61	6.1%	3.81	
Baseball	97–98	51,351	289	22	0.43	2.7%	5.38	50.2*
	98–99	49,207	293	6	0.12	2.0%	1.71	
	99–00	80,215	482	25	0.31	5.2%	7.75	
Gymnastics	97–98	277	1	0	0	0%	0	0
	98–99	221	0	0	0	0%	0	
	99–00	1,179	8	0	0	0%	0	

Note: IDR = Incidence Density Ratio.
[a]Total concussions divided by total athlete exposures. [b]Of all reported injuries, percentage of injuries that were concussions. [c]Ratio comparing games to practice-injury rates. [d]Chi-squares comparing games to practices.
*Statistically significant at $p = .01$.

Football

Data were collected in the sport of football for 361 teams (an average of 120 per year) during the 3-year period. Concussions accounted for 6.7% of all reported injuries during fall practice, 8.8% during football games, and 5.5% during spring football practices over the 3-year period. Players were found to have a 10 times (IDR 10.54) greater risk of suffering a concussion during football games than practices over the 3-year period. Results revealed that football players in the 1999–2000 season reported a significantly higher number of concussions than for the 1997–1998 ($\chi^2 = 36.20$) and 1998–1999 football seasons ($\chi^2 = 23.5$). Results also indicated a significantly higher number of concussions during the 1999–2000 practice season when compared to the 1997–1998 practice season ($\chi^2 = 16.25$). Interestingly, game injury rates almost doubled from the 1997–1998 (2.32) to the 1999–2000 football (4.15) seasons (see Table 1).

Ice Hockey

During the 3-year period, data for ice hockey were recorded for 95 teams (an average of 32 per year). One hundred and twenty-six players sustained a concussion during the 3-year study. Of all the injuries suffered by ice hockey players, concussions accounted for 6.3% of practice injuries and 10.3% of game injuries. Ice hockey players were found to be at a 15.5 times greater risk for suffering a concussion during games than during practice sessions.

Soccer

In men's soccer, 267 teams (an average of 89 per year) were analyzed during the 3-year period. One hundred and twenty-three concussions occurred during the 3 years, with game concussions accounting for 7.0% and practice concussions accounting for 1.7% of all the reported injuries. Male soccer players were at a

Table 2. *Male Practice Concussions*

Sport	Year	Total Practices	Total Number of Injuries	Total Concussions	Concussion Injury Rates[a]	Percentage of Concussions[b]
Football	97–98	637,698	2,415	145*	0.23	6.0%
	98–99	640,871	2,683	180	0.28	6.7%
	99–00	846,300	3,949	284*	0.34	7.2%
Hockey	97–98	69,795	152	12	0.17	7.9%
	98–99	52,369	108	5	0.1	4.6%
	99–00	78,757	172	10	0.13	5.8%
Spring	97–98	113,711	1,274	78	0.67	6.1%
Football	98–99	50,619	529	39	0.77	7.4%
	99–00	83,213	1,004	67	0.66	6.7%
Wrestling	97–98	92,782	661	17	0.18	2.6%
	98–98	51,381	323	20	0.35	6.2%
	99–00	83,213	604	28	0.31	4.6%
Basketball	97–98	118,905	424	16	0.14	3.8%
	98–99	164,607	693	31	0.19	4.5%
	99–00	140,637	569	22	0.16	3.9%
Lacrosse	97–98	76,246	282	11	0.14	3.9%
	98–99	56,201	215	4	0.07	1.9%
	99–00	74,115	223	14	0.19	6.3%
Baseball	97–98	127,623	316	10	0.08	3.2%
	98–99	130,988	284	9	0.07	3.2%
	99–00	213,674	413	9	0.04	2.2%
Soccer	97–98	127,013	535	10	0.08	1.9%
	98–99	77,769	369	8	0.11	2.2%
	99–00	106,241	440	4	0.04	0.9%
Gymnastics	97–98	3,897	5	0	0	0%
	98–99	3,265	7	0	0	0%
	99–00	9,867	60	0	0	0%

[a]Total concussions divided by athlete exposures. [b]Of all reported injuries, percentage of injuries that were concussions.
*Statistically significant at $p = .01$.

21.9 times greater risk of suffering a concussion during games than practices. Male soccer players' IDR tripled from the 1998–1999 (12.82) season to the 1999–2000 season (39.00).

Data were collected in the sport of women's soccer for 288 teams (an average of 96 per year) during the 3-year period. One hundred and ninety-two concussions were reported during the 3 years. The IDR was 16.7 times higher for games than practice sessions. Of all the injuries suffered by female soccer players, concussions accounted for 11.4% for games and 2.4% for practice.

Lacrosse

One hundred and nineteen teams were analyzed in men's lacrosse (an average of 40 per year) during the 3-year period. Eighty concussions were reported during the 3-year study. Of all injuries sustained during men's lacrosse, 4.0% represented practice concussions and 10.1% represented game concussions. Injury rates for concussions in games were 13.32 times higher than practice sessions.

Women's lacrosse reported data on 112 teams (an average of 37 per year) during the 3-year period. Of all injuries sustained during women's lacrosse, 5.3% represented practice concussions and 13.9% represented game concussions. The IDR was 6.3 times higher during games than practices.

Wrestling

Results revealed that, out of 143 wrestling teams (an average of 47 per year), 121 concussions were sustained over the 3 years. The IDR was 8.7 over the 3 years. However, the IDR was 18.1 for the 1997–1998 season and then dropped significantly to 2.2 in the next season ($\chi^2 = 12.64$). Concussions account for 6.6% during matches and 4.5% during practices.

Table 3. *Female Game Concussions*

Sport	Year	Total Games	Total Number of Injuries	Total Concussions	Concussion Injury Rates[a]	Percentage of Concussions[b]	IDR[c]	Chi-Square[d]
Lacrosse	97–98	8,762	75	12	1.37	16.0%	3.26	23.74*
	98–99	7,122	52	7	0.98	13.5%	9.80	
	99–00	8,531	58	7	0.82	12.1%	5.86	
Soccer	97–98	24,981	454	51	2.04	11.2%	14.57	478.83*
	98–99	22,934	430	47	2.05	10.9%	18.64	
	99–00	27,167	497	60	2.21	12.1%	17.00	
Basketball	97–98	29,413	233	16	0.54	6.9%	2.35	45.33*
	98–99	38,174	349	30	0.78	8.6%	4.11	
	99–00	28,992	262	26	0.89	9.9%	3.87	
Softball	97–98	26,834	143	9	0.34	6.3%	2.27	0.24
	98–98	44,280	197	10	0.23	5.1%	2.56	
	99–00	75,355	365	28	0.37	7.7%	2.64	
Field Hockey	97–98	11,065	78	3	0.27	3.8%	1.59	8.11*
	98–99	4,770	43	5	1.05	11.6%	10.5	
	99–00	11,278	65	4	0.35	6.2%	7.00	
Volleyball	97–98	24,904	124	5	0.2	4.0%	4.00	6.05
	98–99	24,482	90	4	0.16	4.4%	8.00	
	99–00	35,203	151	6	0.17	3.9%	1.89	
Gymnastics	97–98	8,903	34	1	0.11	0.3%	0.84	0.002
	98–99	822	12	0	0	0%	0	
	99–00	2,083	23	0	0	0%	0	

Note: IDR = Incidence Density Ratio.
[a]Total concussions divided by total athlete exposures. [b]Of all reported injuries, percentage of injuries that were concussions. [c]Ratio comparing games to practice injury rates. [d]Chi-squares comparing games to practices.
*Statistically significant at $p = .01$.

Table 4. *Female Practice Concussions*

Sport	Year	Total Practices	Total Number of Injuries	Total Concussions	Concussion Injury Rates[a]	Percentage of Concussions[b]
Lacrosse	97–98	33,342	158	14	0.42	8.9%
	98–99	31,048	82	3	0.1	3.6%
	99–00	37,765	149	5	0.14	3.4%
Basketball	97–98	104,872	497	24	0.23	4.8%
	98–98	140,817	617	26	0.19	4.2%
	99–00	108,480	495	25	0.23	5.1%
Softball	97–98	45,291	165	7	0.15	4.2%
	98–99	76,076	229	7	0.09	3.1%
	99–00	129,155	345	17	0.14	4.9%
Field Hockey	97–98	41,340	130	7	0.17	5.4%
	98–99	19,398	59	2	0.1	3.4%
	99–00	42,016	138	3	0.05	2.2%
Soccer	97–98	87,442	457	12	0.14	2.6%
	98–99	77,286	472	9	0.11	1.9%
	99–00	100,855	507	13	0.13	2.6%
Volleyball	97–98	60,179	203	3	0.05	1.5%
	98–99	31,130	337	1	0.02	0.3%
	99–00	88,875	369	8	0.09	2.2%
Gymnastics	97–98	31,006	224	4	0.13	1.8%
	98–99	9,253	45	0	0	0%
	99–00	19,829	136	1	0.05	0.7%

[a]Total concussions divided by total athlete exposures. [b]Of all reported injuries, percentage of injuries that were concussions.

Basketball

Men's basketball reported data on 372 teams (an average of 124 per year) during the 3-year period. One hundred and eighteen athletes suffered a concussion, with concussions accounting for 4.1% of all the injuries sustained during practices and 5.0% during games. Results indicated game injury rates doubled from the 1997–1998 season (0.29) to 1999–2000 season (0.61). However, injury rates were not significant over the 3 years.

Women's basketball reported data on 376 teams (an average of 125 per year) during the 3-year period. Female basketball players suffered a total of 147 concussions. Concussions accounted for 4.7% of all the injuries sustained during practices and 8.5% during games. Women basketball players are at a 3.4 times higher risk of suffering a concussion during a game situation than a practice session. Results revealed a gradual increase in game injury rates from the 1997–1998 season (0.54) to the 1999–2000 season (0.89).

Field Hockey

Data were collected in women's field hockey for 104 teams (an average of 35 per year) during the 3-year period. Twenty-four concussions were reported over the 3-year period, with an IDR of 6.4. Concussions accounted for 3.7% of all injuries suffered during practices and 7.2% during games.

Softball

Data were collected in the sport of softball for 331 teams (an average of 110 per year) during the 3-year period. IDR was 2.5 times greater for softball games than for practices. A total of 78 concussions were reported during the 3-year study. Practice concussions accounted for 4.1% of all injuries, while game concussions accounted for 6.4% of all injuries.

Baseball

Baseball reported 337 teams (an average of 112 per year) with an IDR 3.8 times greater for games than practices. Eighty-one concussions were reported during the 3-year study. Results found 2.9% of all practice injuries were concussions and 4.2% of all game injuries were concussions.

Volleyball

Data were analyzed in volleyball for 304 teams (an average of 101 per year) during the 3-year period. Twenty-seven concussions were reported for the 3-year study. Of all the injuries reported, concussions accounted for 1.3% during practices and 4.1% during games. Volleyball players are at a 3.8 times greater risk of sustaining a concussion during a game situation than a practice session.

Gymnastics

Data were collected in the sport of women's gymnastics for 49 teams (an average of 16 per year) during the 3-year period. Women's gymnastics reported four practice concussions during the 1997–1998 season and one concussion during the 1999–2000 season. Only one competition concussion was reported during the 1997–1998 season, with no other concussions reported for the next 2 years. Results revealed no concussions were sustained in men's gymnastics for 12 teams (an average of 4 per year) during the 3-year period.

Discussion

The purpose of this study was to examine the incidence and prevalence of concussions among 15 different intercollegiate sports during the 1997–1998 season to the 1999–2000 season. During this 3-year study, concussions accounted for 6.2% of all reported injuries. Powell and Barber-Foss (1999) reported that mild traumatic brain injury accounted for 3.9% of all injuries suffered in 10 high school sports. The differences found in our study may be attributed to sample population (high school versus college), grading scale of concussions, and the design of the study. Furthermore, our study included ice hockey, women's and men's lacrosse, and spring football, which may have contributed to the higher concussion rate.

The differences in concussion rates in all male sports except gymnastics were found to be significant between games and practices, whereas female soccer, basketball, lacrosse, and field hockey were also found to be significant between games and practices. Female athletes from all seven sports were found to be at a lower risk for suffering concussions during practice sessions than the eight male sports. However, women were found to be at a greater risk for suffering concussions during games than men. Further research is needed to determine why women are suffering a greater number of concussions during games but not practices. One possible explanation is female athletes may be practicing at a lower intensity level relative to their game level intensity than male athletes. Alternatively, there may be neuropsychological differences in the susceptibility to concussions among women.

Concussions in Football Players

Of all the sports, football was found to have the highest number of concussions suffered during both practices and games. Our results indicate 8.8% of all football players are at risk for sustaining a concussion during games. This is in agreement with Barth et al. (1989), who indicated 7.7% were, and McCrea et al. (1998), who reported that 5.8% of all football injuries are concussions during a single season.

Athletes at Risk for Suffering a Concussion

Athletes at the highest risk for suffering a concussion are those participating in football, ice hockey, wrestling, men's and women's soccer, and men's and women's lacrosse. A possible explanation may be the nature of each sport. For example, football and ice hockey are considered contact sports in which contact is an expected and often desirable part of the game. Although soccer and women's lacrosse do not involve intentional collisions between players, incidental collisions frequently occur as a result of heading. Given the current findings, it appears important that researchers continue to track these athletes and develop strategies to reduce the number of concussions sustained yearly.

Athletes who participate in men's and women's gymnastics, baseball, softball, and volleyball are at the lowest risk for suffering a concussion. A possible explanation may be the safety standards or the low risk of contact. Gymnastics is considered a high-risk sport but not for concussions. Gymnasts land on soft mats or into foam pits, which cushion the blow or force to the head. Baseball and softball players wear a helmet to protect them from head injuries. Volleyball players rarely make head-to-head contact with each other or the floor.

Concussions in Male Athletes

Of all the male sports, ice hockey players suffered the greatest percentage of concussions during game situations (10.3%). These results contradicted Tegner and Lorentzon (1996), who reported 6.5% of elite hockey players sustained a concussion during league play and concluded that 20% of elite ice hockey players will endure one concussion during their career. When you consider injury rates, football players suffered the greatest number of concussions in relation to AEs. Furthermore, football was the only sport to report statistical significance between years. Football players during the 1999–2000 season reported a significantly higher number of concussions during games compared to the 1997–1998 and 1998–1999 seasons. Football players also experienced a significantly greater number of concussions during the 1999–2000 practice season than the 1997–1998 practice season.

Concussions in Female Athletes

Women's soccer was found to have the highest injury rate and IDR among all women's sports. Although women's lacrosse was found to have the highest inherent risk of sustaining a concussion during a game situation (13.9%), female lacrosse players sustain very few injuries compared to other female sports. This would suggest that female lacrosse is a relatively safe sport; however, the percentage of injuries classified as concussions is considerably higher than in other female sports. Recently, there has been considerable debate among coaches and safety committees as to whether helmets should be worn to protect lacrosse players from head injuries (Brown, 2001). Brown (2001) argued that if female lacrosse players wear safety equipment, athletes will become more aggressive, making the game more dangerous.

Reporting Concussions

High-profile concussions focus on professional hockey and football players. Recently, the NHL and National Football League implemented baseline neuropsychological assessment of all players (Lovell & Collins, 1998). Once an athlete has sustained a concussion, he or she completes the neuropsychological test battery at the following postinjury intervals: 24 hr, 5 days, and 10 days (Macciocchi, Barth, Alves, Rimel, & Jane, 1996). To help evaluate cognitive deficits, neuropsychological baseline tests should be implemented in middle school, high school, and collegiate athletes, especially for football and ice hockey players. Furthermore, epidemiological studies should be conducted on middle school and high school athletes to determine injury rates on concussions. Recently, researchers are becoming more effective in reporting IDRs; however, there still remains work to be done with classifying athletes with concussions and implementing a screening maintenance plan.

Limitations of This Study

There are several limitations to this study. First, there is no common definition, grading scale, or measure of severity of concussions for the NCAA ISS. As a result, what one athletic trainer or physician may report as a Grade 1 concussion may be classified by another healthcare provider as a Grade 2 concussion. However, it should be noted that all grades of concussions in this study were represented in the overall percentages of concussions sustained by athletes.

Another limitation to this study is the evaluation of AEs. The NCAA ISS reports an AE as an athlete participating in one game or practice where she or he is exposed to the possibility of athletic injury. However, an athlete who plays a 45-sec hockey shift during a game is reported as participating in one game. Another hockey player who played 21 min of the game is also represented as exposed to one game. As a result, time played is not considered in the definition of AE.

Conclusion

Concussions accounted for 6.2% of all reported injuries during this 3-year study. Female athletes from all seven sports were found to be at a lower risk for suffering concussions during practice sessions than the eight male sports. However, female athletes were found to be at a greater risk for suffering concussions during games than male athletes. Concussions continue to be on the rise for football players, whereas those participating in ice hockey, men's and women's lacrosse, men's and women's soccer, women's basketball, and wrestling are all at risk for suffering a concussion.

Future research is needed to establish yearly injury trends to determine which athletes are at a greater risk for acquiring a concussion. Research is also needed to evaluate and implement strategies to reduce the number of concussions sustained yearly by collegiate, high school, and middle school athletes. Further empirical studies are needed to establish baseline neuropsychological assessments for all collegiate, high school, and middle school sports to help aid in the return to play criteria.

This article reviewed important epidemiological characteristics of college athletes. Neuropsychologists who are practicing in this area should familiarize themselves with these data to understand the base rates for concussions in the sport that they may be assisting with. Trends over time and gender differences are important aspects of the landscape of concussions of athletes. Neuropsychologists should understand the complexity of concussion rates in intercollegiate athletics in order to become informed and competent consultants when dealing with a college student population.

References

American Medical Association. (1966). *Subcommittee on classification of sports injuries: Standard nomenclature of athletic injuries.* Chicago: Author.

Barnes, B., Cooper, L., Kirkendall, D., McDermott, T. P., Jordan, B., & Garrett, W. (1998). Concussion history in elite male and female soccer players. *American Journal of Sports Medicine, 26,* 433–438.

Barth, J., Alves, W., Ryan, T., Macciocchi, S., Rimel, R., Jane, J., et al. (1989). Mild head injury in sports: Neuropsychological sequelae and recovery of function. In H. S. Levin, H. M. Eisenberg, & A. L. Benton (Eds.), *Mild head injury* (pp. 257–275). New York: Oxford University Press.

Boden, B., Kirkendall, D., & Garrett, W. (1998). Concussion incidence in elite college soccer players. *American Journal of Sports Medicine, 26,* 238–241.

Brown, J. (2001, May). Checking in on girls youth lacrosse rules. *Lacrosse Magazine,* pp. 26–30.

Bruce, D. A., Schut, L., & Sutton, L. N. (1982). Brain and cervical spine injuries occurring during organized sports activities in children and adolescents. *Clinics in Sports Medicine, 1,* 495–514.

Buckley, W. (1988). Concussions in college football. *Journal of the American Medical Association, 16*(1), 51–56.

Cantu, R. C. (1996). Guidelines for return to contact sports after a cerebral concussion. *The Physician and Sportsmedicine, 14*(10), 75–83.

Cantu, R., & Voy, R. (1995). Second impact syndrome. *The Physician and Sportsmedicine, 23*(6), 27–34.

Congress of Neurological Surgeons. (1966). Committee on Head Injury Nomenclature: Glossary of head injury. *Clinical Neurosurgery, 12,* 386–394.

Delaney, S., Lacroix, V., Leclerc, S., & Johnston, K. (2000). Concussions during the1997 Canadian Football League season. *Clinical Journal of Sport Medicine, 10,* 9–14.

Evans, R. W. (1994). The postconcussion syndrome: 130 years of controversy. *Seminars in Neurology, 14,* 32–39.

Fekete, J. (1968). Severe brain injury and death following minor hockey accidents. *Canadian Medical Association Journal, 99,* 1234–1239.

Gerberich, S., Priest, J., Boen, J., Straub, P., & Maxwell, R. (1983). Concussion incidences and severity in secondary varsity football players. *American Journal of Public Health, 73,* 1370–1375.

Kelly, J. P. (1995). Concussion. In J. S. Torg. (Ed.). *Current therapy in sportsmedicine* (3rd ed.). Philadelphia: Mosby.

Kelly, J., Nichols, J., Filey, C., Lillehei, K., Rubinstein, D., & Kleinschmidt-DeMasters, B. (1991). Concussion in sports: Guidelines for the prevention of catastrophic outcome. *Journal of the American Medical Association, 266,* 2867–2869.

Lorentzon, R., Wedren, H., & Pietila, T. (1988). Incidence, nature and causes of ice hockey injuries: A three year prospective study of a Swedish elite ice hockey team. *American Journal of Sports Medicine, 16,* 392–396.

Lovell, M., & Collins, M. (1998). Neuropsychological assessment of the college football player. *Journal of Head Trauma Rehabilitation, 13,* 9–26.

Macciocchi, S., Barth, J., Alves, W., Rimel, R., & Jane, J. (1996). Neuropsychological functioning and recovery after mild head injury in collegiate athletes. *Neurosurgery, 39,* 510–514.

Maroon, J., Lovell, M., Norwig, J., Podell, K., Powell, J., & Hartl, R. (2000). Cerebral concussion in athletes: Evaluation and neuropsychological testing. *Neurosurgery, 47,* 659–672.

McCrea, M., Kelly, J., Kluge, J., Ackley, B., & Randolph, C. (1997). Standardized assessment of concussion in football players. *Neurology, 48,* 586–588.

McCrea, M., Kelly, J., Randolph, C., Kluge, J., Bartolic, E., Finn, G., et al. (1998). Standardized assessment of concussion (SAC): On-site mental status evaluation of the athlete. *Journal of Head Trauma Rehabilitation, 13*(2), 27–35.

McCrory, P., & Berkovic, S. (1998). Concussive convulsions: Incidence in sport and treatment recommendations. *Sports Medicine, 25,* 131–136.

Miettinen, O. S. (1976). Estimatability and estimation in case-referent studies. *American Journal of Epidemiology, 103,* 226–235.

National Collegiate Athletic Association. *NCAA Injury Surveillance System for academic year 1997–2000.* Indianapolis, IN: Author.

Powell, J., & Barber-Foss, K. (1999). Traumatic brain injury in high school athletes. *Journal of the American Medical Association, 282,* 958–963.

Quality Standards Committee, American Academy of Neurology. (1997). Practice parameter: The management of concussion in sports (summary statement). *Neurobiology, 48,* 1–5.

Saunders R. L.,& Harbaugh, R. E. (1984). The second impact in catastrophic contact-sports head trauma. *Journal of the American Medical Association, 252,* 538–539.

Tegner, Y., & Lorentzon, R. (1996). Concussion among Swedish elite hockey players. *British Journal of Sports Medicine, 30,* 251–255.

Thurman, D., & Guerrero, J. (1999). Trends in hospitalization associated with traumatic brain injury. *Journal of the American Medical Association, 282,* 954–957.

Original submission May 1, 2002
Accepted August 9, 2002

Applied Neuropsychology
2003, Vol. 10, No. 1, 23–30

The Neuropsychology of Repeated 1- and 3-Meter Springboard Diving Among College Athletes

Eric A. Zillmer

Department of Athletics, Drexel University, Philadelphia, Pennsylvania, USA

This study examined the neuropsychological effects of repeated springboard diving. It was hypothesized that the impact velocity, which can range from 20 to 30 mph, and accompanying deceleration in the water may lead to concussions and affect the diver's cognitive function. Six varsity National Collegiate Athletic Association Division 1 springboard divers participated in the study. Each diver performed a total of 50 practice dives from either the 1- or 3-m springboard. After each set of 10 dives, the participants were immediately evaluated at poolside using the Symbol Digit Modalities Test, the Stroop Color Word Test, and the Trail Making Test B. Baseline testing revealed, consistent with their athletic specialty, clear neurocognitive strengths among the divers on tests sensitive to proprioception, motor speed, and visual–spatial organization. Results from the serial assessments indicated no detectable neuropsychological deficits among competitive divers compared to baseline testing. Skilled diving at the collegiate level appears to be a safe sport and water appears to present the perfect medium for gradual deceleration. More studies, however, are warranted for 5-, 7.5-, and 10-m platform diving since the impact velocity of the diver from these heights is higher.

Key Words: sports-related concussion, springboard diving, neuropsychological assessment

Many sports involve speed and the potential for collision. Repeated blows to the head, like those occurring in boxing and football, and potentially in springboard diving, have been associated with the likelihood for concussions or mild traumatic brain injury (MTBI) in the athlete (Barth, Freeman, Broshek, & Varney, 2001). The symptoms of MTBI have been documented most frequently with motor vehicle accidents. There are, however, analogous situations involving the acceleration and deceleration of the head in the context of competitive sports. Frequent head impact can place the athlete at risk for MTBI even when experiencing relatively minor concussive forces to the head. In some cases this has resulted in excessive dizziness, difficulty in concentrating, and neurocognitive changes in the athlete (Echemendia & Julian, 2001).

The sport of springboard diving can be dangerous to the participant for those reasons. Many diving wells warn the recreational diver that serious head and neck injuries can result from improper diving. Slips, falls, hitting the board, diving into shallow water, whiplash, and colliding with other swimmers in the water have all led to a high rate of injuries, including those of the neck and head. In some instances, these have even resulted in death. The risk of injury has led to prohibitive insurance rates for public swimming pools that have diving boards. As a result, many recreational swim clubs have removed 3-m boards from their premises and have implemented strict safety regulations for the use of 1-m springboards. There are, however, no statistics available on accidents related to diving boards only. Additionally, shallow water accidents are also classified as diving accidents, inflating the statistics of diving-related accidents further.

I would like to acknowledge Barbara Holda, Jennifer Wiser, Rhonda Freeman, Tania Giovanetti, Amy Gordon, Kaira Hayes-Miller, Terri Horowitz, Linda Meisenhelder, Burton Weiss, and Michael Colis for assisting with the data collection. I particularly appreciate Frank Ferrone's input regarding the physics of diving. I would also like to thank former diving coach Beth Bauer, current diving coach Larry May, the Drexel University diving team, as well as the former intercollegiate athletic director Johnson Bowie for their support.

Requests for reprints should be sent to Eric A. Zillmer, 3141 Chestnut Street, Department of Athletics, Drexel University, Philadelphia, PA 19104, USA. E-mail: zillmer@drexel.edu

A further potential for injury may be the repeated exposure of the brain to the impact of headfirst entries into the water. Depending on the height of the dive and the level of skill, divers experience varying degrees of force as they make contact with the surface of the water and decelerate. The impact velocity and accompanying deceleration that divers experience may result in concussive forces associated with a decreased capacity to concentrate and process complex information. Deceleration in the water among divers is variable and dependent on the stopping distance, that is, the distance from water entry until the end of vertical descent. For example, a diver who enters the water at 22 mph (or 9.9 m/s) from a 3-m springboard, would decelerate 13.4 m/s^2 or approximately 1.5 g for a 12-ft stopping distance. If the diver would complete his or her descent in the water at a 6-ft stopping distance, the deceleration would be twice as strong, 26.8 m/s^2 or 3 g. Ten-meter tower diving may be particularly hazardous given the great forces as the diver enters the water at average speeds of over 30 mph. There are currently, however, no known studies on the neuropsychology of springboard or platform diving that have examined the potential for cumulative and acute effects on the brain.

As in many other sports, competitive springboard divers start in childhood, often as young as 5 years old. Organized competitions from the 1-m board, including dives with a headfirst entry, can start as early as age 6. Around age 10, divers compete from the 3-m board with almost exclusively headfirst entry and year-round meets. During adolescence, club divers often start 5- and 7.5-m platform diving, and some divers compete and practice on 10-m towers. Competitive divers train several hours a day, performing as many as 50 dives per training session. Practices can be as frequent as six times per week and are typically year-round. In college, diving is regulated by the National Collegiate Athletic Association (NCAA) to facilitate the academic progress of the student-athlete. Practice is seasonal (i.e., 5 to 6 months) and restricted to 20 hr per week. By the time a competitive diver has completed his or her college career, he or she has completed a total of over 100,000 dives.

This study examined the cumulative and acute neuropsychological effects of repeated 1- and 3-m springboard diving among college athletes to determine the degree, if any, of brain injury as reflected objectively using neuropsychological procedures. An additional goal of this study was to calculate the exact forces acting on each diver in contrast to other studies on sports-related concussions that infer such information or use self-reports.

Method

Participants and Materials

Six varsity NCAA Division 1 divers (average age 21 years, 4 female) from an east-coast university participated in the study. All were administered a comprehensive neuropsychological battery for the purpose of establishing a neurocognitive baseline and for evaluating any neuropsychological deficits that may be related to the cumulative effects of springboard diving. The tests employed in this study included the Halstead-Reitan Neuropsychological Test Battery (Reitan & Wolfson, 1993) and the Wechsler Adult Intelligence Scale–Revised (WAIS–R; Wechsler, 1981). In addition, and of particular importance to the study, was the employment of measures that were sensitive to complex, sustained attention and higher-order problem solving, two areas of cognitive function that have repeatedly been shown to be impaired in individuals with head injuries (Zillmer & Spiers, 2001). Three tests of complex attention were selected based on their construct validity as sensitive measures of attention and concentration and new problem solving, as well as their suitability for serial administration at poolside (Lezak, 1995). These assessment techniques included the Trail Making Test B from the Halstead-Reitan Neuropsychological Battery, the Symbol Digit Modalities Test (Smith, 1982), and the Stroop Color Word Test (Golden, 1976).

Procedures

Within 3 weeks of the baseline evaluation, the following experimental procedure was performed during a practice session at the university's swimming and diving facility. Two groups (i.e., one for the 1-m and the other for the 3-m springboard) of 3 divers each performed 50 practice dives. All participants attempted the same type of dive for each set of 10 dives. Each diver completed, in order, 10 forward dives, 10 backward dives, 10 reverse dives, 10 inward dives, and 10 forward dives with one-half twist. These dives are also known as required or basic dives, and all involve a headfirst entry. The dives are relatively easy maneuvers for accomplished divers. Thus, some divers added a pike or tuck position to the dives to increase the difficulty of the dive.

After each set of 10 dives, all divers were assessed immediately at poolside tables using the Trail Making Test B, the Digit Symbol Modalities Test, and the Stroop Color Word Test, by one of three available psychometricians. In addition, all dives were timed to measure the impact velocity as the divers made contact with the water. This was accomplished by measuring the time elapsed from the top of the dive, using the center of body mass, until entry into the water. The center of body mass was considered to be midchest in men and upper abdomen in women. The average time for each diver at the 1-m height and the 3-m height was multiplied by the acceleration of gravity or 9.8 m/sec^2 according to the following formula: velocity = the product of acceleration and time ($v = gt$). Maximum and minimum impact velocities for each diver were then calculated. Deceleration in the water was separately measured using an underwater observation window by timing the descent of each diver beginning from the water entry to the end of vertical descent. The average descent times were then divided into the average velocities to calculate deceleration ($a = v/t$).

Results

Neuropsychological Baseline Testing

Test scores of the expanded Halstead-Reitan battery can be examined in Table 1. The Average Impairment Rating was used as a measure of overall neuropsychological functioning and ranged from 0.2 to 0.5 for the 6 divers (i.e., within normal limits). WAIS–R Full Scale IQ (FSIQ) scores fell within the average to high-average range of intellectual abilities (i.e., range = 102–109, M FSIQ = 107). Variability between the individual subscales of the WAIS–R for both verbal and performance subtests was also within normal limits. Interestingly, three of the divers obtained higher Performance IQs (PIQs), compared to their Verbal IQs (VIQs), of 9 points or more. The average PIQ–VIQ split was +6.2 (range = −3 to +23; cf. Zillmer, Ball, Fowler, Newman, & Stutts, 1991, discusses PIQ–VIQ splits). This suggests that the divers, on average, performed better on items requiring perceptual motor speed than on tasks necessitating verbal comprehension skills. Neuropsychological test results indicated that the cognitive efficiency of all 6 participants was consistently above a T score of 40 on tests of complex attention and new problem solving (see Table 1). Taken together, baseline neuropsychological test results revealed average, and in some cases, above average, cognitive functioning for all 6 divers. Significant strengths were found on neuropsychological procedures sensitive to proprioception, eye-hand coordination, visual-spatial organization, and processing speed.

Thus, there was little evidence for a consistent pattern of deficits that could be associated with a "chronic diving syndrome."

Velocity and Deceleration Results

Results (see Table 2) indicated an average impact velocity of 7.58 m/s for the 1-m board and 9.54 m/s for the 3-m board. Maximum impact velocity was 9.21 m/s (1-m) and 12.94 m/s (3-m), corresponding to approximately 21 and 29 mph maximum impact speed, respectively. The average deceleration was 9.06 m/s^2 for the 1-m board and 16.28 m/s^2 for the 3-m board, which corresponds to approximately 1 to 2 g. During deceleration, divers were observed to avoid impact with the 13-ft deep diving pool bottom by curving away from vertical descent into horizontal motion after entering the water. Deceleration was most rapid for divers who curved into horizontal motion soonest. The profile of deceleration varied considerably because of the diver's underwater technique employed to enter the water with proper body alignment and minimal splash. Skilled divers often change their body position underwater to achieve a more consistent entry with less splash by using a forward somersault save or a backward knee save (see Figure 1), resulting in increased deceleration values.

Neuropsychological Testing Poolside

The average time interval between each of the 5 diving sets was 21 min. Each diver performed 10 dives and was administered poolside three neuropsychological test procedures within that time interval prior to the next set of 10 dives. The findings from serial administration of the neuropsychological measures indicated average to above average performances with marked practice effects occurring over the five trials of testing (see Figures 2–4). Among the 72 possible serial comparisons (i.e., 6 participants × 4 serial trials × 3 procedures = 72), only 8% of the trials showed no improvement compared to the trial before. No differences were found in the performance profiles of divers using the 1- or 3-m board.

Discussion

In this study, the cumulative and acute effects of springboard diving were evaluated using neurocognitive testing to determine the degree, if any, of brain injury as

Table 1. *Neuropsychological Test Scores for Six National Collegiate Athletic Association Division 1 Springboard Divers*

| | Diver #[a] | | | | | | | | | | | |
| | 1[b] | | 2[c] | | 3[d] | | 4[e] | | 5[f] | | 6[g] | |
	Scaled Score[h]	T-Score[i]	Scaled Score	T-Score	Scaled Score	T-Score	Scaled Score	T-Score	Scaled Score	T-Score	Scaled Score	T-Score
Intellectual Functioning (WAIS–R)												
Information	12	51	08	28	11	46	12	47	08	32	10	39
Digit Span	06	32	10	45	13	55	12	52	10	45	13	52
Vocabulary	10	39	10	39	10	39	10	39	12	48	10	46
Arithmetic	11	39	08	33	13	58	15	60	12	54	13	58
Comprehension	10	40	11	43	08	32	12	47	11	43	13	51
Similarities	14	57	09	35	14	57	09	35	12	48	08	31
Picture Completion	09	47	09	39	11	52	11	48	11	52	09	43
Picture Arrangement	07	35	12	56	12	56	14	64	10	47	13	56
Object Assembly	12	61	14	61	12	53	10	53	10	45	13	57
Digit Symbol	12	47	12	51	15	60	11	47	16	64	08	30
Verbal IQ	102	43	95	32	109	47	109	45	105	43	103	43
Performance IQ	102	44	118	59	118	59	109	51	114	55	100	40
Full Scale IQ	102	38	105	42	114	51	109	47	109	47	103	42
Average Impairment Rating	.5	59	.2	78	.2	75	.2	77	.2	77	.2	78
Abstract Reasoning, Complex Attention												
Category Test (Short-form errors)	30	43	21	48	06	71	08	64	15	52	08	64
Trail Making Test A (sec.)	13	75	23	51	20	53	15	66	22	50	17	63
Trail Making Test B (sec.)	36	66	53	52	43	56	30	71	38	62	46	58

	C1	C2	C3	C4	C5	C6	C7	C8	C9	C10	C11	C12
Seashore Rhythm (correct)	28	52	27	49	27	48	27	48	28	52	28	52
Speech Sounds Perception (errors)	02	56	02	57	03	52	00	75	06	42	02	49
TPT Localization	02	56	10	57	08	63	04	44	03	41	09	75
SDMT[i] (Correct)	67	1.5[j,k]	71	2.5[j]	82	2.0[j]	55	0.0	75	1.0[j]	85	2.0[j]
Stroop Word (Correct)	89	40	107	50	126	59	109	50	119	55	106	49
Stroop Color (Correct)	65	40	73	45	101	64	70	44	91	57	84	53
Stroop Color Word (Correct)	41	46	40	45	70	65	46	51	65	70	44	51
Motor Speed and Coordination												
Finger Oscillation DH	47.6	50	51.4	44	49.8	54	57.5	55	52	58	47.4	51
Finger Oscillation NDH	43.4	50	42.6	39	40	46	50.6	50	47.2	58	42	51
Grip Strength in kg DH	31.5	52	54	49	34.5	57	50	44	26.5	46	35.5	56
Grip Strength in kg NDH	27.5	51	54.2	54	27.5	51	47	49	29.5	51	34.5	55
TPT dominant min. per block	.72	40	.41	55	.44	51	.29	66	.21	77	.6	42
TPT non-dominant min. per block	.75	34	.21	63	.18	66	.2	66	.18	65	.47	43
TPT both hands min. per block	.21	51	.1	69	.14	59	.16	55	.18	53	.17	56
Memory												
TPT Memory	02	37	10	70	09	58	08	47	09	58	09	59

Note: WAIS–R = Wechsler Adult Intelligence Scale–Revised; TPT = Tactual Performance Test; SDMT = Symbol Digit Modalities Test; DH = dominant hand; NDH = nondominant hand. [a] All divers had right-hand dominance (from Lateral Dominance Examination). [b] Twenty-one-year-old female with 14 years of education. [c] Twenty-year-old male with 13 years of education. [d] Twenty-one-year-old female with 15 years of education. [e] Twenty-two-year-old male with 15 years of education. [f] Twenty-three-year-old female with 14 years of education. [g] Nineteen-year-old female with 13 years of education. [h] Age-corrected scaled scores. [i] Education and age corrected *T*-scores from Heaton, Grant, and Matthews (1991) except where otherwise noted. [j] Normalized T-scores from Wetzel and Boll (1987). [k] Age-corrected deviation units from the mean (Smith, 1991).

Table 2. *Velocity and Declaration Data*

	Diver #	Gender	Age	Average v (m/s)	v min (m/s)	v max (m/s)	Max Impact Velocity (mph)	Deceleration (m/s²)
1-m s/b	1	Female	21	7.15	4.50	8.72	19.50	8.61
	2	Male	20	8.13	6.37	9.21	21.00	9.80
	3	Female	21	7.45	5.98	8.82	20.00	8.76
	4	Male	22	10.19	7.06	12.94	29.00	20.80
3-m s/b	5	Female	23	9.02	5.19	11.27	25.00	12.36
	6	Female	19	9.41	5.10	12.50	28.00	15.68

Note: v = velocity; s/b = springboard.

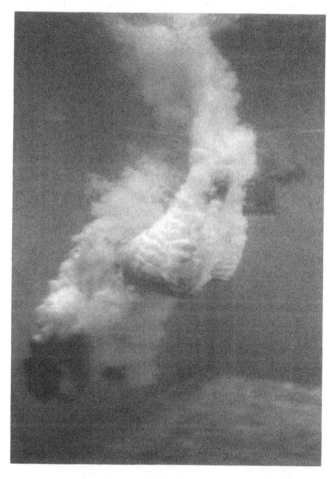

Figure 1. Divers entering the water often experience different turbulences and markedly different rates of deceleration. This diver is performing a backward knee save to accomplish a vertical entry from the 3-meter springboard.

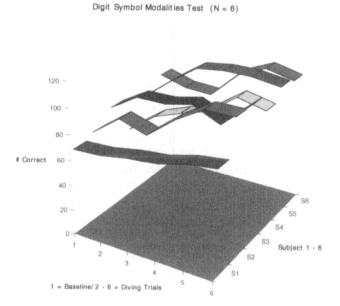

Figure 2. Performance curves on the Digit Symbol Modalities Test.

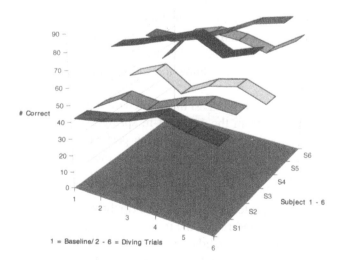

Figure 3. Performance curves on the Stroop Color Word Test.

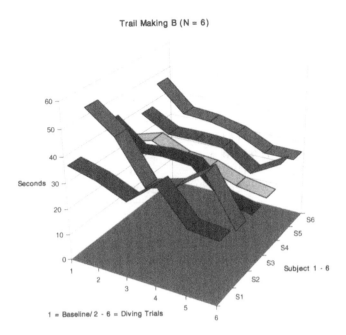

Trail Making B (N = 6)

Figure 4. Performance curves on Trail Making Test B.

reflected in objective neuropsychological procedures. These results indicated no detectable neuropsychological deficits that can be attributed to the effects of competitive college springboard diving. In fact, results from neuropsychological testing demonstrated that skills, which require the positioning and movement of the limbs and motor speed, were clear relative strengths among the six NCAA Division 1 divers. That competitive divers would show a keen sense for body positioning, spatial orientation, and balance should come as no surprise since proprioception, visualization, and eye-hand coordination are all necessary for skilled diving. On tests of complex and sustained concentration only 8% of all trials resulted in a worse performance than the previous trial. This deterioration appears negligible and may be related to the fact that the tests were not administered in a standard testing room but at poolside, or perhaps it is attributable to fatigue or test-ceiling effects. Alternatively, this finding may also represent normal variation.

These results suggest that skilled diving at the collegiate level from the 1- and 3-m springboard is a safe sport and that water presents the perfect medium for gradual deceleration. Coincidentally, the technique involved in competitive diving may protect the head. Particularly in skilled diving, the hands of the divers serve as a protection to provide a rip through which the splash, and, indirectly, the impact on the head, is minimized. This is a standard technique that divers use for aesthetic reasons to create an air pocket by which the body can enter into the water with little or no splash

(see Figure 5). Most experts on diving agree that the palm of the hand should make contact with the water first to initiate a good entry. The hand should be held horizontally so the diver should feel impact with the water dead center on the palm of the lead hand. During entry, the head is kept aligned with the body and movement of the head is taught to be avoided (O'Brien, 1992). It is thus likely that this technique of entering the water protects the head by placing disproportional stress on the hands, wrists, and shoulders of the diver thus avoiding impact and rotational stress on the head. As a result, it is the wrists and shoulders where divers are most susceptible to injury. In addition, lower back injuries are common as the result of improper alignment during water entry.

The results of this study are limited to 1- and 3-m springboard diving among college athletes. Further studies with elite divers are warranted, since they accumulate many more dives, particularly from 5-, 7.5-, and 10-m platforms, where the impact velocity can be consistently over 30 mph. In fact, 10-m tower diving among elite athletes is often associated with injuries to the eardrum, thumb-caps, wrists, shoulders, as well as welts and even broken noses related to the considerable forces experienced at entry. Platform divers often report that the repeated impact of diving from

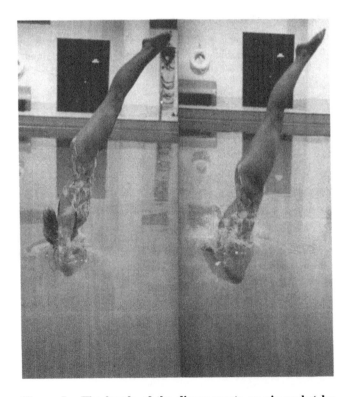

Figure 5. The hands of the divers create an air pocket by which the body can enter into the water with little or no splash indirectly minimizing the impact on the head.

the tower is so substantial that most platform divers practice no more than 30 dives in a day and then stay away from the platform for two days to let their bodies heal. Joints become stiff. Shoulders separate. This is not a sport for the timid. (Montville, 1995, pp. 57–58)

In view of such reports, the neuropsychological effects of platform diving and cliff diving should be evaluated particularly in light of several elite athletes retiring from the sport because of excessive dizziness. Such studies would add to an understanding of whether similar injuries are primarily peripheral, that is related to the vestibular system, or primarily "central," that is, caused by impairment in neuropsychological processing. In addition, further studies with high school divers, who may be less skilled and may have a greater potential for injury because of their age, are indicated.

This study was conducted to educate professionals about the potential for neurocognitive impairment in college divers and to provide reassurance for the relative safety of the sport at the college level. The small number of participants ($N = 6$), however, suggests that these results should be interpreted with caution. More comprehensive studies should be considered particularly research involving younger divers and increased heights.

References

Barth, J. T., Freeman, J. R., Broshek, D. K., & Varney, R. N. (2001). Acceleration-deceleration sports-related head injury: The gravity of it all. *Journal of Athletic Training, 36,* 253–256.

Echemendia, R. J., & Julian, L. J. (2001). Mild traumatic brain injury in sports: Neuropsychology's contribution to a developing field. *Neuropsychology Review, 11,* 69–88.

Golden, C. (1976). A group version of the Stroop Color and Word Test. *Journal of Personality Assessment, 39,* 386–395.

Heaton, R. K., Grant, I., & Matthews, C. G. (1991). *Comprehensive norms for an extended Halstead-Reitan battery: Demographic corrections, research findings, and clinical applications.* Odessa, FL: Psychological Assessment Resources.

Lezak, M. D. (1995). *Neuropsychological assessment* (3rd ed.). New York: Oxford University Press.

Montville, L. (1995, August). Vexed by vertigo. *Sports Illustrated,* 55–61.

O'Brien, R. (1992). *Diving for gold: Basic to advanced springboard and platform skills.* Champaign, IL: Leisure Press.

Reitan, R. M., & Wolfson, D. (1993). *The Halstead-Reitan neuropsychological test battery: Theory and clinical interpretation* (2nd ed.). Tucson, AZ: Neuropsychology Press.

Smith, A. (1982). *Symbol Digit Modalities Test* (manual revised 1982). Los Angeles: Western Psychological Publishers.

Wechsler, D. (1981). *WAIS–R manual.* New York: Psychological Corporation.

Zillmer, E. A., & Spiers, M. V. (2001). *Principles of neuropsychology.* Belmont, CA: Wadsworth.

Zillmer, E. A., Ball, J. D., Fowler, P. C., Newman, A. C., & Stutts, M. L. (1991). Wechsler verbal-performance IQ discrepancies among psychiatric inpatients: Implications for subtle neuropsychological dysfunction. *Archives of Clinical Neuropsychology, 6,* 61–71.

Original submission May 1, 2002
Accepted August 9, 2002

Applied Neuropsychology
2003, Vol. 10, No. 1, 31–41

Recency and Frequency of Soccer Heading Interact to Decrease Neurocognitive Performance

Frank M. Webbe and Shelley R. Ochs

School of Psychology, Florida Institute of Technology, Melbourne, Florida, USA

This study investigated the role of heading recency interacting with heading frequency in determining neuropsychological deficits associated with heading the ball during soccer play. Sixty-four high-ability male soccer players ages 16 to 34 completed the California Verbal Learning Test (CVLT), the Trailmaking Test, the Paced Auditory Serial Addition Test (PASAT), the Facial Recognition Test, the Rey-Osterrieth Complex Figure, and the Shipley Scales. Heading recency interacted with heading frequency, such that players with the highest self-reported estimates of heading who also experienced heading within the previous 7 days scored significantly lower on CVLT, Shipley, Trailmaking, and PASAT than other combinations of heading and recency. Although strict ball-to-head contacts could not be isolated as sufficient to cause this interaction, these results increase the weight of evidence that heading behavior is problematic for causing at least transient cognitive impairment.

Key words: soccer, traumatic brain injury, athletic participation, neuropsychology, sport psychology

The sport of soccer extends its reach throughout the world. Perhaps because the requisite equipment is minimal and inexpensive, or possibly because of the basic simplicity of the major act of kicking a ball, soccer vies each year for the title of the most played game and most watched sport in the world. Injuries in soccer have been noted to occur at a moderate-to-high rate. For example, recent National Collegiate Athletic Association (NCAA) injury statistics show that the game injury rates for men's soccer were 20.1 per 1,000 athlete exposures (AEs; by comparison, rates for football were 37 injuries per 1,000 AEs). For collegians, nearly 10% of all soccer injuries were head injuries (Latest fall sports study, 2001), with concussion being the dominant form of head injury in both college and high-

school soccer players (Powell & Barber-Foss, 1999). Players may hit their heads on the ground or against goal posts, but the major source of head injuries is interplayer collision (Frenguelli, Ruscito, Bicciolo, Rizzo, & Masserelli, 1991). Adding to the risk of head injury from accidental collisions or rough play, players also use their head intentionally to strike the ball as an integral part of the game. Heading creates considerable excitement among fans, particularly when players leap into the air and compete with each other for possession of the ball. These attempts also increase the risk of head-to-head or other head-related collisions, in addition to creating the ball-to-head blows. Tysvaer and Lochen (1991); Abreu, Templer, Schuyler, and Hutchinson (1990); Matser, Kessels, Jordan, Lezak, and Troost (1998); and Witol and Webbe (in press) have all reported depressed neuropsychological performance for players who head the ball very frequently in comparison to players whose heading behavior is less frequent. In accounting for these results, Matser et al. (1998) and Witol and Webbe (in press) have regarded heading events as accumulations over a lifetime of many subconcussive blows to the head. Moreover, the level of deficit observed has typically been similar to that seen in acute cases of mild traumatic brain injury (MTBI) with American collegiate football players

We are grateful to Karl Evans, Becky Ochs, and Sherry Ochs for assistance with data collection. Preparation of this article was supported by a sabbatical leave grant from the Florida Institute of Technology to the first author and by the Brain Injury and Sport Concussion Institute of the University of Virginia Health Sciences Center, J. T. Barth, Director. A preliminary report of these data was presented at the 20th Annual Meeting of the National Academy of Neuropsychology, Orlando, FL (November, 2000).

Requests for reprints should be sent to Frank M. Webbe, School of Psychology, Florida Institute of Technology, 150 W. University Blvd., Melbourne, FL 32901, USA. E-mail: webb@fit.edu

(Barth et al., 1989; Macciocchi, Barth, Alves, Rimel, & Jane, 1996). In contrast to these studies, other research has concluded that known history of concussion is sufficient to account for any neuropsychological deficit that occurs within the context of soccer play and that heading is irrelevant (Green & Jordan, 1998; Kirkendall, Jordan, & Garrett, 2001). And indeed, even though the literature on soccer injuries is studded with occasional anecdotal accounts of wooziness and confusion following an intense heading event (e.g., Mathews, 1972), only one study has reported systematically on the temporal relationship among heading events with neuropsychological performance. Putukian, Echemendia, and Mackin (2000) administered a brief neuropsychological battery to a sample of college-level players before and after 90-min practice sessions that included about 20 min of heading work. No neurocognitive effects of the heading intervention either between groups or within participants were demonstrated. Unfortunately, a highly significant practice effect for both heading and comparison groups across the testing sessions in this pre-post design could have easily obscured a heading effect if one was present. Moreover, the qualitative differences between practice and game headings are pronounced, both in terms of unanticipated jostling at the time of ball-head impact, and in the intensity of the behavior.

The purpose of this study was to assess the role of recent heading activity in determining neuropsychological performance in a sample of soccer players who were grouped based on how recently they had headed the ball in games and practice. Moreover, the contribution of heading frequency was also studied in interaction with recency so as to describe more fully conditions under which neurocognitive weakness might occur.

The seeming capriciousness with which heading relationships have been reported to occur or not occur in previous studies might suggest that heading is a relatively weak causal agent in comparison to other determinants of impaired neurologic and neurocognitive performance. Another possibility for the variability may be that heading interacts with other factors in additive or multiplicative ways in causing impairments. Hence, the analysis of *recency* of heading activity interacting with frequency as a mediating factor in depressed neuropsychological performance was pursued here. Studies of mild head injury in college football players (Macciocchi et al., 1996) and reviews of post-concussion syndrome generally (PCS; Bernstein, 1999) have reported that it takes about a week for acute concussion effects to subside in the majority of cases.

A smaller subset of mild head-injury patients requires considerably longer to regain premorbid cognitive levels (Reitan & Wolfson, 1999). These studies indicate that somatic and cognitive symptoms of distress may persist even after concussion assessment test data have returned to baseline or at least begun such a recovery. Thus, it is quite possible that the inconsistent effects within and between soccer-heading studies might reflect an underlying process such as duration of post-concussion effects related to (a) time since previous play and (b) current heading activity. Since neuropsychologists will consult on cases involving soccer players and other athletes at-risk for brain trauma, it is important for them to consider that athletes who have not reported recently with concussion may yet have unresolved and even unknown concussion symptoms.

Method

Participants

Sixty-four male soccer players from across central Florida volunteered to participate. Most were starting players, and they represented seven high-level teams from high school, college, premier development, and professional leagues. The high school and college teams had contended for or won their state (Florida High School Athletic Association) or national association (NCAA) titles. The premier development team was a perennial contender for championship in the United Soccer Leagues, and the professional team was a franchise of Major League Soccer. Twenty currently active male athletes with minimal experience in football, hockey, soccer, or lacrosse (and none at all in the past 5 years) served as a comparison group. The comparison athletes engaged mainly in running, cycling, basketball, and baseball. For the soccer players, the participants' mean age was 21.09 ($SD = 4.31$), with a range from 16 to 34. The comparison athletes' average age was 21.20 ($SD = 4.35$), with a range from 16 to 34. Education for soccer players was 13.73 ($SD = 2.42$) years and for comparison athletes was 14.00 ($SD = 2.43$) years.

Participants were excluded if they (a) admitted any current recreational use of illicit drugs, (b) admitted to present or past heavy use of alcohol (greater than two drinks per day), (c) had suffered serious head trauma, (d) had been diagnosed with a learning disability or attention deficit or hyperactivity disorder. These criteria were implemented to reduce sources of variability that could result in neuropsychological impairment regardless of current soccer or heading activity. Of the 64 total participants, 4 were goalkeepers who reported no heading. Their data are not included in the analyses.

The nature and procedure of the study was described in detail to all prospective participants. Volunteers completed a consent form before participating in any data collection, as prescribed by the Florida Tech Institutional Review Board for Human Experimentation. The final sample of participants consisted of those who volunteered and who also met the inclusion criteria. Approximately 60 players who were invited to participate declined, most citing insufficient time in their schedules to accommodate the testing. Only a handful of players disqualified themselves based on exclusion criteria.

Instruments

Prior to testing, a structured interview was conducted in which the participants answered questions regarding demographic, medical, and sport history including heading practices. Specific information was elicited concerning head injuries, however minor, and any somatic and cognitive complaints related to heading.

During the testing session, participants were administered a battery of six standardized neuropsychological tests. The tests and rationale for use were as follows. The California Verbal Learning Test (CVLT) was used due to its sensitivity to generic memory problems and learning deficits caused by head trauma (Delis, Kramer, Kaplan, & Ober, 1987; Lezak, 1995, p. 447). The score on the 5th learning trial, the total score for the 5 learning trials with list A, the score for recall following a long (20-min) delay, and the number of perseverations are reported. The Rey-Osterrieth Complex Figure Test (ROCF; Rey, 1941, sections of which were translated in Corwin & Bylsma, 1993) was used for its sensitivity to visual memory and visuospatial impairments (Taylor, 1969). The Trailmaking Test, Parts A and B, has been shown to differentiate brain injury groups from other groups and is sensitive to the effects of brain injury (Lezak, 1995, p. 383; Reitan, 1955). The Shipley Institute of Living Scale was used in this study both to obtain estimates of Wechsler Adult Intelligence Scale–Revised Full Scale IQ scores, and as a broad measure of verbally based conceptual performance (CQ; Zachary, 1986). The short form of the Facial Recognition Test (FRT; Benton & Van Allen, 1968) represented a nonverbal test of brain function, particularly of right parietal lobe functioning (Levin, Hamsher, & Benton, 1975). The Paced Auditory Serial

Addition Test (PASAT; Gronwall, 1977) was included due to its sensitivity in detecting subtle decrements in information processing skills, which are usually associated with minor head injuries (Gronwall & Wrightson, 1981; Bernstein, 1999). Thus, a total of 16 dependent measures represented this battery. A participant's performance on a neuropsychological measure was considered to be impaired when a score at least 2 *SD* below the mean was obtained.

Procedure

All participants were tested without distraction in quiet, comfortable settings—either in the living room of their homes or in a testing laboratory that was furnished similar to a home. Participants appeared motivated, and the players especially approached testing as they might a match. Interview and testing was usually completed within 2 hr. Four primary examiners were used, and they followed standardized procedures of administration. All tests were scored by S. Ochs. The sequence of test administration was as follows: CVLT, ROCF (copy), Trailmaking Test Parts A and B, Shipley (CQ), CVLT (Delayed Recall), Shipley (IQ), ROCF (Delayed Recall), FRT, and PASAT.

Players were also questioned concerning when they had last played or practiced soccer, and whether they headed the ball on those occasions. This allowed a measure of playing and heading recency, which was used as the basis for forming groups for further analysis of recency effects. Specifically, a recency group was formed of 39 players who had played or practiced and headed the ball within the past 7 days. The nonrecency group ($n = 19$) had neither played nor practiced (nor headed the ball) within 7 days of testing. Seven days was selected as a representative duration at which previous studies have concluded that most sequelae of MTBI have resolved for most players (Collins et. al., 1999; Macciocchi et al., 1996). Fortuitously, there was about a 2-week lull in the playing history of most participants after the 7-day cutoff, which eliminated any near overlap in the recency groups.

The heading measure. As in previous studies of soccer heading, the participant's self-reported estimate of heading was used as the primary measure or the basis for deriving other metrics (Jordan, Green, Galanty, Mandelbaum, & Jabour, 1996; Matser et al., 1998; Witol & Webbe, in press). Each soccer player provided a subjective report of his heading practices by answering the following items during the structured interview: (a) the number of times he headed the ball in a typical game and practice, (b) whether he considered himself to be a header, (c) his frequency of heading compared to other players, and (d) his frequency of heading the ball according to different positions played. To describe current heading practices, participants were divided into four heading groups: comparison (Group 1, no heading), low (Group 2, 0–5 times per game), moderate (Group 3, 6–10 times per game), and high (Group 4, more than 10 times per game). A cumulative heading measure was created by multiplying the current heading estimate by the years of experience in competitive soccer. This latter measure assumes a constant number of games and practices per year. The cumulative groups were formed by keeping together the 20 comparison participants to form Group 1 and forming Groups 2 through 4 by creating break points for the three remaining quartiles in the distribution of the cumulative heading measure.

Results

The results are organized according to the following progression that addresses factors shown in previous studies to differentiate soccer players' neuropsychological test performance: (a) player demographics and histories, (b) differences in neuropsychological test scores between soccer players and comparison athletes and comparisons across heading groups, (c) comparison of percentages of individual neurocognitive tests in an impaired range across heading categories, (d) symptom differences based on heading frequency, (e) role of concussion history in possibly accounting for depressed neurocognitive function, (f) interaction of heading recency with heading frequency.

Demographics and player histories. The soccer participants in this sample were highly skilled players who had been performing at advanced competitive levels for at least 5 years. The demographics of the sample are presented in Table 1; details are provided for group (soccer vs. control), category of play (high school, college, amateur, and professional), and team. Table 1 also shows the number of years of soccer experience, the average number of playing minutes in games for the most recent season, whether the player considered himself to be a header of the ball, and the history of concussion due to (a) heading the ball, (b) other head trauma while playing soccer, or (c) head injury unrelated to soccer play. The total concussion column is not a simple sum of the preceding three, since some players experienced multiple concussions in the various settings.

The soccer and control group means for age and education did not differ. Of the seven teams from which participants were recruited, the intent of selection was to assess the starting field players, and, in fact, a majority of the starters volunteered. Team C had the smallest ratio of starters at just 50%, whereas 93% of Team F participants reported that they were starters (13 of 14). Since only 10 can truly start, a post hoc interview revealed that some players did not generally travel to away games. Therefore, this team had a starting line-up that differed by several players between home and away games. Table 1 also shows the average playing time, which typically relates to starting versus substitute role. Most players represented here played

Table 1. *Sample Demographics by Group, Category, and Team*

	n	Age	Education Years	Starters	Years Played	Playing Time (min)	Is a Header	Source of Concussion			
								Heading	Soccer	Other	Total
High School	13	16.9	10.1	100%	8.9	75.8	62%	8%	0%	23%	31%
Team A	7	17.1	10.4	7	12.0	75.0	5	1	0	2	3
Team B	6	16.5	9.8	6	5.2	76.7	3	0	0	1	1
College	30	19.8	13.7	73%	12.7	63.0	40%	3%	33%	23%	50%
Team C	11	20.3	14.3	10	13.4	76.8	5	0	2	2	4
Team D	10	19.8	13.3	5	11.9	39.0	2	1	2	2	4
Team E	9	19.11	13.4	7	12.9	69.4	5	0	6	3	7
Premier Amateur (F)	14	25.1	16.2	93%	19.4	86.8	43%	0%	36%	7%	43%
Professional (G)	7	26.6	15.6	100%	19.1	83.6	71%	14%	57%	14%	57%
Total Soccer	64	21.09	13.73	88%	14.09	72.58	31 (48%)	3 (5%)	19 (30%)	12 (19%)	29 (45%)
Comparison	20	21.20	14.00								0 (0%)

the majority of the maximum game duration (80 min for high school, 90 min for all others). Nearly half (48%) of the players identified themselves to be headers. In the vernacular of the game, this implies that they seek out opportunities to head the ball and consider themselves to be skilled in the mechanics of directing the ball with the head.

Since complete medical data covering entire careers were not readily available, the determination of previous concussions was based on player response to the personal history questions on concussion, loss of consciousness (LOC), and treatment by a physician or hospital as a result of head injury. More than 30% of the players reported suffering concussion (with or without LOC) without consulting a physician (although they may have consulted a trainer, a possibility that was not fully assessed). No comparison athletes reported incidents of head injury, concussion, or LOC.

Forty-five percent of all players had suffered concussion, with 11 of them (18%) admitting to multiple concussions. Three of the players reported concussion following an incident of heading the ball; 19 reported concussion after other soccer events such as contact with another player; 12 players had suffered concussion in head trauma contexts other than soccer. The mean duration for all instances of LOC due to concussion was slightly more than 2 min, although the median value was 15 sec. A Chi-square test revealed no significant differences in concussion across the categories of play, $\chi^2(3, n = 60) = 1.823, p = .612$.

Comparison of soccer players to comparison athletes to heading groups. As Table 2 shows, soccer players exhibited weaker performance on 14 of the 16 dependent measures than did the nonsoccer athletes; however, these differences were mostly small and not significant except for CVLT perseverations, the 2.0 interval of the PASAT, and the Shipley IQ.

The role of heading was analyzed by grouping players into low, medium, and high heading categories based upon their self report of current heading practices as described in Procedure. Players who reported the highest frequency of heading the ball generally had the weakest performance; however, the group differences were small, and none were statistically significant. Use of the cumulative heading measure produced similar findings.

Incidence of test scores in impaired range. From an applied, clinical standpoint, more critical than average differences across groups are results that demonstrate impaired performance for individual participants. Table 3 shows the percentages of player test scores in an

Table 2. *Means and Standard Deviations for Soccer and Comparison Groups*

	Comparison[a]		Soccer[b]		
	M	**SD**	**M**	**SD**	**t**
CVLT Total	57.25	8.91	54.03	7.56	-1.575
Trial 5	13.50	2.25	12.65	1.77	-1.729
Long Delay	12.35	2.83	11.53	2.31	-1.289
Perseveration	3.60	2.45	6.38	4.51	2.625**
FRT	46.10	3.64	47.08	3.93	.985
ROCF Copy	33.70	1.98	33.20	2.46	-.824
Delay	23.05	5.10	22.49	5.47	-.401
PASAT Total	166.00	29.08	152.20	34.82	-1.581
2.4 s	49.45	7.45	44.96	9.64	-1.851
2.0 s	47.85	7.07	43.25	8.63	-2.131*
1.6 s	39.00	9.19	37.02	9.94	-.778
1.2 s	29.70	8.05	26.96	10.09	-1.091
Shipley IQ	110.25	4.94	105.42	9.23	-2.277*
CQ	103.85	7.97	108.10	11.05	1.584
Trailmaking					
Part A	20.15	5.79	21.53	6.55	.840
Part B	43.15	11.24	46.11	13.92	.860

Note: CVLT = California Verbal Learning Test; FRT = Facial Recognition Test; ROCF = Rey-Osterrieth Complex Figure Test; PASAT = Paced Auditory Serial Addition Test. All values are raw scores except for the Shipley Scales, which are normalized.
[a]$n = 20$. [b]$n = 60$.
*$p < .05$. **$p < .01$.

impaired range across groups. Participants in all groups (including the control athletes) exhibited impaired performance on one or more of the measures. The percentages for the soccer players were higher than for the comparison athletes, though no difference across heading groups was observed. When the test batteries were examined for individual players, as would be done in a clinical evaluation, 5 participants, all soccer players, scored in an impaired range on three or more of the six instruments. Of these 5, 1 came from the low-heading group, and 2 each came from the moderate- and high-heading groups. No comparison athletes were so impaired. The CVLT and ROCF measures exhibited several scores in an impaired range even with the comparison athletes. No problems or irregularities in administration were detected. Only soccer players exhibited impaired scores on FRT, PASAT, and Trailmaking.

Somatic and cognitive complaints. We also asked the players to report on four somatic (blurred vision, dizziness, headache, numbness or tingling) and three cognitive complaints related to heading (confusion, poor

Table 3. *Percentage of the 16 Assessment Measures in an Impaired Range for the Heading and Comparison Groups*

		Heading[a]		
	Comparison[b]	Low[c]	Moderate[d]	High[e]
CVLT Total	10%	16%	18%	13%
Trial 5	20%	16%	35%	33%
Long Delay	20%	21%	18%	8%
Perseveration	0	0	6%	4%
FRT	0	11%	12%	21%
ROCF Copy	10%	16%	0	13%
Delay	10%	11%	0	4%
PASAT Total	0	0	0	13%
2.4 s	0	13%	6%	21%
2.0 s	0	0	0	4%
1.6 s	0	0	0	0
1.2 s	0	0	0	13%
Shipley IQ	0	5%	12%	4%
CQ	5%	5%	6%	8%
Trailmaking Part A	0	5%	0	0
Part B	0	5%	6%	0
Group Totals	5%	8.5%	7.8%	8.8%

Note: CVLT = California Verbal Learning Test; FRT = Facial Recognition Test; ROCF = Rey-Osterrieth Complex Figure Test; PASAT = Paced Auditory Serial addition Test.
[a]$n = 60$. [b]$n = 20$. [c]$n = 19$. [d]$n = 17$. [e]$n = 24$.

concentration, and memory loss). These represent categories of symptoms that commonly predominate on concussion and postconcussion checklists (Guskiewicz, 2001; Macciocchi et al., 1996). Most players reported that they rarely or never were bothered by these symptoms. A greater percentage of players in the moderate- (13.2%) and high- (12.5%) heading groups reported somatic complaints than did those in the low frequency category (7.8%). Only 2 players reported any cognitive complaints, 1 in the low, and 1 in the moderate group. Somatic and cognitive complaints also were evaluated based on history of LOC. Players who had a history of concussion were bothered by somatic and cognitive complaints no more than the no-concussion players (11.4% vs. 9.5%).

Role of head injury history. Because the presence of a history of head injury from any origin may be a significant factor in controlling variance in neurocognitive test scores, and since history of head injury was known for these participants (see Table 1), the player group was split based on history of concussion. Test scores were examined for the two resulting groups of soccer players (concussion and no concus-

sion) and the comparison athletes. History of concussion was not predictive of differences in neurocognitive performance among soccer players. The comparison athletes generally performed a bit better, though not significantly so.

Interaction of frequency of heading with recency of play. The simple comparison of the means of test scores for players who had or had not played or practiced within the past 7 days resulted in no significant differences on any measures. Indeed, the group means were nearly identical. However, factorial analysis of variance (ANOVA) showed that recent heading interacted with frequency such that players with the highest estimates of game heading, who also played soccer and experienced heading within the previous 7 days, scored significantly lower than other groups on the CVLT Trial 5 and Total scores, the Shipley CQ, Trailmaking Parts A and B, and the PASAT 2.4 Trial. These comparisons are shown in Table 4. The frequent headers who played most recently also exhibited the weakest (though not significantly so) performance of any of the groups in five of the nine remaining measures. Representative graphic portrayals of these results for Shipley CQ, Trailmaking, CVLT Total, and PASAT Total appear in Figure 1.

A breakdown of who played recently showed that the premier and professional players all had played recently, whereas the high school and college players were about evenly divided. (College and high school seasons had ended and some players had begun play with club teams). This resulted in significant differences in both age and education; both were greater for the recency players ($M_{age} = 22.56$; $M_{educ} = 14.49$) than the nonrecency players ($M_{age} = 19.16$; $M_{educ} = 12.89$), $t(56) = 2.994$, $p < .004$ and $t(56) = 2.556$, $p < .013$, respectively. There was, however, no interaction either of education, $F(2, 52) = .719$, $p = .492$, or age, $F(2, 52) = 1.170$, $p = .318$, between the recent play-frequent heading cell with the nonrecent play-frequent heading cell. Nonetheless, since education can impact the neurocognitive tests used here (more so than age for the age ranges of this study), the factorial ANOVAs were all repeated with education as a covariate. No changes in outcome occurred for any of the comparisons. Finally, since concussion history and acute concussion incidence have been widely implicated in soccer players' cognitive functioning in past studies, the recency by frequency interaction groups were evaluated with respect to these factors. There was an equal distribution of players in the recent and nonrecent groups who had experienced concussion,

Table 4. *Interaction of Heading Recency with Heading Frequency (Means Only)*

Played in Last 7 Days	Low		Moderate		High		F
	Yes[a]	No[b]	Yes[a]	No[c]	Yes[d]	No[e]	
CVLT Total	54.45	51.25	56.09	52.80	52.82	60.33	3.023*
Trial 5	12.82	12.75	13.09	12.20	11.94	14.00	3.316*
Long Delay	11.82	10.25	12.64	10.40	11.53	12.50	2.310
Perseveration	5.09	7.13	6.82	8.80	6.88	4.67	1.156
FRT	46.36	44.63	49.36	45.60	47.53	47.83	1.120
PASAT Total	163.00	142.57	173.90	144.40	140.06	151.40	1.388
2.4 s	49.25	39.48	50.85	43.59	40.39	48.32	3.905*
2.0 s	46.96	43.04	46.90	40.52	40.16	44.87	1.540
1.6 s	40.77	35.12	44.47	33.88	34.29	33.85	.862
1.2 s	29.72	23.46	34.14	25.81	24.25	27.00	1.184
ROCF Copy	32.95	32.87	34.45	33.80	32.67	33.00	.149
Delay	21.59	21.06	25.68	21.60	21.76	24.08	1.274
Shipley CQ	109.73	103.13	106.82	109.40	106.00	119.33	3.826*
IQ	108.64	104.13	107.55	105.40	102.41	108.17	1.780
Trailmaking Part A	18.36	23.44	19.91	20.12	24.24	19.13	3.472*
Part B	42.82	51.81	41.91	46.20	47.82	37.50	3.661*

Note: CVLT = California Verbal Learning Test; FRT = Facial Recognition Test; PASAT = Paced Auditory Serial Addition Test; ROCF = Rey-Osterrieth Complex Figure Test. All values are raw scores except for the Shipley Scales, which are normalized.
[a]$n = 11$. [b]$n = 8$. [c]$n = 5$. [d]$n = 17$. [e]$n = 6$.
*$p < .05$. **$p < .01$.

$\chi^2(1, n = 58) = 0.225$, $p = .781$. Six players reported concussion within the current season; all 6 were in the recent-play group and were divided equally among the low-, moderate-, and high-heading groups.

Discussion

These results supported the notion that very recent heading of moderate-to-high frequency related to weaker neurocognitive performance. These results were clearest for the CVLT, the Shipley CQ, Trailmaking Parts A and B, and the PASAT. Although the Shipley was administered primarily to document, via the IQ estimate, that groups were similar in general intelligence, the lower CQ score is consistent with a slight cognitive decline. The lower CVLT total score implies some difficulty in verbal learning, possibly implicating conceptual difficulties as well. In addition to suggesting the presence of brain injury, the depressed Trailmaking scores also imply difficulty in planning and attention. The lowered PASAT score suggests the possibility of reduction in information processing speed and impaired divided-attention ability.

In analyzing the role of recency of play, it was found that the players in the recency group were older and better educated. They generally scored somewhat higher on the tests shown in Figure 1 than the nonrecency players at the low and moderate levels of heading behavior. The separation of the scores of the recent-frequent heading players from the non-recent-frequent heading players was, in many instances, due both to depressed scores of the recent group and to seemingly elevated scores of the nonrecent group (e.g., CVLT Total) relative to the other combinations of the interaction (as was shown graphically in Figure 1). Since education and age did not differ significantly between these two cells of the interaction, it seems likely that the acute effects of frequent heading depressed otherwise high functioning in this group of players.

The basic comparison of neuropsychological performance of soccer players versus control athletes, as well as the comparison in performance across the heading groups showed, at most, a weak heading effect. Although these results contrast with other studies that have used similar methods but have shown some significant differences in neuropsychological performance (between soccer players and other athletes,

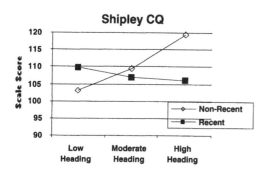

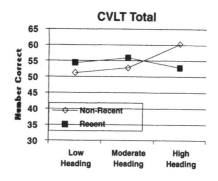

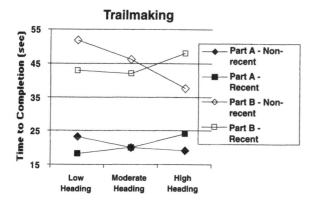

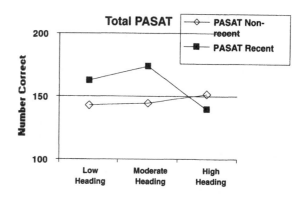

Figure 1. Interaction of heading recency and heading frequency. Shown are scale (Shipley CQ) or raw scores (California Verbal Learning Test Total, Trailmaking Parts A & B, and Paced Auditory Serial Addition Test Total) for groups of players who did (Recent) or did not play (Nonrecent) within the previous 7 days across three categories of heading.

Matser et al., 1998, and between heading frequency groups, Witol & Webbe, in press), they are similar to studies that have found no effects of heading (Jordan et al., 1996). Similar to Witol and Webbe (in press), somatic complaints and the percent of impaired test scores were greater for the soccer players who reported the most heading activity.

Some studies have also estimated cumulative heading behavior over a lifetime and found that more heading was linked to greater neurocognitive deficits (Abreu et al., 1990; Matser et al., 1998; Matser, Kessels, Lezak, Jordan, & Troost, 1999; Witol & Webbe, in press). In this study, no significant or strong effect was found for lifetime heading on neuropsychological performance. Comparisons of the estimates of current heading and the estimates of cumulative heading resulted in no difference in outcomes. Possible reasons for this seeming conflict with other studies that used similar methodologies were that (a) the players in this study really were not meaningfully separated by age and total soccer experience, and (b) the variability in estimation of heading in interaction with

the lack of variability in age and experience created too much within-group variance to reveal a heading effect if one were present. Although the age range varied from 16 to 34, 72% of the players were aged 19 to 24. Although player estimation of heading appeared to be an adequate measure in this and other studies, the normal variability that characterizes this measure may hinder finding anything other than a very strong between-group statistical effect. Strong effects have not been the norm in previous heading studies. Instead, most studies found considerable variability in test scores within groups, and reported that at least as many neurocognitive tests have failed to differentiate between soccer and control groups, or among heading groups, as have succeeded in doing so (e.g., Matser et al., 1998; Matser et al., 1999; Witol & Webbe, in press).

There appears to be no disagreement with the contention that soccer players are at risk for head injury, and that neurocognitive performance may be at least transiently depressed by acute head trauma (Jordan et al., 1996; Kirkendall et al., 2001). Considerable disagreement persists, however, regarding any relationship between (a) length of soccer career or (b) the role of heading (particularly ball-to-head contacts) as causal agents producing neurologic and neurocognitive decline or chronic deficit. Kirkendall et al. (2001) and Green and Jordan (1998) both argued against any such roles in their reviews of the research. Matser et al. (1998; Matser et al., 1999) and Witol and Webbe (in press) pointed to consistencies in their results that differentiate level of neurocognitive impairment based on heading frequency over years played. Clearly, a major difficulty in all such research is differentiating ball-to-head contacts as causative for injury within a context where traumatic head injuries can occur due to more obvious agents such as collisions with fixed objects or others' body parts. Some researchers (Jordan et al., 1996) adopted the perspective that since heading was not the obvious cause of concussion, it was not a candidate for causing neurocognitive deficits. In this study, 3 players reported that an incidence of heading resulted in concussion accompanied by brief LOC (< 10 sec). In addition to Mathews' (1972) classic and oft-cited portrayal of "footballer's migraine" in discussing heading after effects, more recent reports of serious neurologic complications related to heading must be taken quite seriously (e.g., Autti, Sipila, Autti, & Salonen, 1997; Kawanishi, Nakayama, & Kadota, 1999). Although acute neurological events due to ball-to-head contacts may be exceptional, they apparently occur with a measurable frequency.

Although these results suggest a different (or at least an additional) mechanism for conceptualizing heading effects than was used in the several studies previously mentioned, they are consistent with Macciocchi et al.'s (1996) findings of acute cognitive impairment following mild head injury in collegiate football players and following concussion generally (Bernstein, 1999). These data suggest that the soccer play of frequent headers may be associated with transient neurocognitive depression not unlike that described for the acute postconcussion period. Moreover, if such a premise is accepted, it helps clarify why some results in previous studies relating heading to neurocognitive deficit have varied so widely. If players are suffering to some extent from a PCS, we can expect there to be considerable variability in intensity, manifestation, and duration of symptoms (Reitan & Wolfson, 1999). Heterogeneity of symptoms within MTBI groups appears to be the rule rather than the exception (Paniak et al., 2002). These results are also consistent with today's theories of the pathophysiology of concussion.

Changes in activity of a cortical glucose metabolic mechanism have been correlated with depressed neurocognitive functioning extending from 24 hr to nearly 10 days postinjury (Hovda et al., 1999). Primary effects were seen in the mesial temporal and frontal lobes. Alteration in the functioning of these brain areas is consistent with the effects shown in the this study.

The 45% concussion incidence is consistent with Barnes et al. (1998), who reported an odds ratio of 50% that elite male soccer players would experience at least one concussion in a 10-year playing career. Moreover, the 18% of players who reported multiple concussions also relates reasonably well to the demographics reported by Barnes and colleagues. However, unlike Barnes et al.'s study of soccer players and Collins et al.'s (1999) study of football players, concussion history did not predict depressed neurocognitive scores. Players who reported concussion within the past 5 years scored similarly to those who had no such history and to the comparison athletes. However, the only players with a concussion in the current year ($n = 6$) all were in the recent play group, which suggests some role of concussion in the depressed test scores.

Barnes et al. (1998) found that headache after heading was the major somatic complaint among 54% of their elite male players (vs. about 30% here). Complaints of dizziness, numbness, and blurred vision occurred much less frequently than headache, though more than reported by players in this study. This hierarchical ordering of symptoms is quite similar to the PCS symptoms that Erlanger et al. (in press) reported for high school and college athletes with recent concussions and may suggest that nondiagnosed concussions were present in Barnes et al.'s (1998) heading sample.

In conclusion, these results support the role of heading as a factor sufficient to depress, at least temporarily, some neurocognitive functioning in some players. At this point, no unambiguous statement can be made concerning what components of heading behavior are causative in this regard and whether such deficits persist over time. Previous studies have clearly documented that risk of head trauma (from collisions and banging heads into objects and bodies) occurring during the act of heading accounts for many instances of neurologic or neurocognitive impairment (Barnes et al., 1998; Boden, Kirkendall, & Garrett, 1998). We cannot say with certainty that either ball-to-head events or head knocks from other sources controlled the present interaction of heading frequency and recency. But regardless of mechanism, players, coaches, trainers, and team physicians need to remain wary of the increased risk factors that appear to be related to frequent heading and to soccer play in general. One conceptualization of these results would suggest that a subset of players routinely exhibit low-level PCS. Any additional insults, either directly from blows to the head or indirectly from bodily collisions and abrupt accelerations might prove problematic for their cognitive functioning (Barth, Freeman, Broshek, & Varney, 2001) or even life threatening (Cantu, 1998). Since athletes are often less than forthcoming about severity of PCS symptoms, it has been recommended previously that baseline assessments be taken before play begins in a season so that removal and return-to-play decisions can be objectively based (Almquist, Broshek, & Erlanger, 2001; Echemendia & Julian, 2001). These data suggest that clinicians would be advised to obtain baseline measurements after at least a week's abstinence from soccer play so as to eliminate any transient cognitive depression. Moreover, in the neuropsychological evaluation, it would be prudent to query players regarding the extent and intensity of their game-related heading.

References

Abreu, F., Templer, D. I., Schuyler, B. A., & Hutchison, H. T. (1990). Neuropsychological assessment of soccer players. *Neuropsychology, 4,* 175–181.

Almquist, J., Broshek, D., & Erlanger, D. (2001). Assessment of mild head injuries. *Athletic Therapy Today, 6,* 13–17.

Autti, T., Sipila, Autti, & Salonen, O. (1997). Brain lesions in players of contact sports. *The Lancet, 349,* 1144.

Barnes, B. C., Cooper, L., Kirkendall, D. T., McDermott, T. P., Jordan, B. D., & Garrett, W. E. (1998). Concussion history in elite male and female soccer players. *The American Journal of Sports Medicine, 26,* 433–438.

Barth, J., Alves, W., Ryan, T., Macciocchi, S., Rimel, R., Jane, J., et al. (1989). Mild head injury in sports: Neuropsychological sequelae and recovery of function. In H. Levin (Ed.), *Mild head injury* (pp. 257–275). New York: Oxford University Press.

Barth, J. T., Freeman, J. R., Broshek, D. K., & Varney, R. N. (2001). Acceleration-deceleration sports-related head injury: The gravity of it all. *Journal of Athletic Training, 36,* 253–256.

Benton, A. L., & Van Allen, M. W. (1968). Impairment in facial recognition in patients with cerebral disease. *Cortex, 4,* 344–358.

Bernstein, D. M. (1999). Recovery from mild head injury. *Brain Injury, 13,* 151–172.

Boden, B. P., Kirkendall, D. T., & Garrett, W. E. (1998). Concussion incidence in elite college soccer players. *American Journal of Sports Medicine, 26,* 238–241.

Cantu, R. C. (1998). Second-impact syndrome. *Clinics in Sports Medicine, 17,* 37–44.

Collins, M., Grindel, S., Lovell, M., Dede, D., Moser, D., Phalion, B., et al. (1999). Relationship between concussion and neuropsychological performance in college football players. *Journal of the American Medical Association, 282,* 964–970.

Corwin, J., & Bylsma, F. W. (1993). Translations of excerpts from Andre Rey's psychological examination of traumatic encephalopathy and P. A. Osterrieth's The Complex Figure Test. *The Clinical Neuropsychologist, 7,* 3–21.

Delis, D. C., Kramer, J. H., Kaplan, E., & Ober, B. A. (1987). *California Verbal Learning Test.* San Antonio, TX: Psychological Corporation.

Echemendia, R. J., & Julian, L. J. (2001). Mild traumatic brain injury in sports: Neuropsychology's contribution to a developing field. *Neuropsychology Review, 11,* 69–88.

Erlanger, D., Kaushik, T., Cantu, R., Barth, J., Broshek, D., Freeman, J., et al. (in press). Symptom-based assessment of concussion severity. *Journal of Neurosurgery.*

Frenguelli, A., Ruscito, P., Bicciolo, G., Rizzo, S., & Masserelli, M. (1991). Head and neck trauma in sporting activities. *Journal of Craniomaxillofacial Surgery, 19,* 178–181.

Gronwall, D. M. (1977). Paced auditory serial-addition task: A measure of recovery from concussion. *Perceptual and Motor Skills, 44,* 367–373.

Gronwall, D., & Wrightson, P. (1981). Memory and information processing capacity after closed head injury. *Journal of Neurology, Neurosurgery, and Psychiatry, 44,* 889–895.

Green, G. A., & Jordan, S. E. (1998). Are brain injuries a significant problem in soccer? *Clinics in Sports Medicine, 17,* 796–809.

Guskiewicz, K. (2001). Concussion in sport: The grading-system dilemma. *Athletic Therapy Today, 6,* 18–27.

Hovda, D. A., Prins, M., Becker, D. P., Lee, S., Bergsneider, M., & Martin, N. A. (1999). Neurobiology of concussion. In J. E. Bailes, M. R. Lovell, & J. C. Maroon (Eds.), *Sports-related concussion* (pp. 12–51). St. Louis, MO: Quality Medical Publishing, Inc.

Jordan, S. E., Green, G. A., Galanty, H. L., Mandelbaum, B. R., & Jabour, B. A. (1996). Acute and chronic brain injury in United States national team soccer team players. *The American Journal of Sports Medicine, 24,* 205–210.

Kawanishi, A., Nakayama, M., & Kadota, K. (1999). Heading injury precipitating subdural hematoma associated with arachnoid cysts. *Neurologia Medico-Chirurgica, 39,* 231–233.

Kirkendall, D. T., Jordan, S. E., & Garrett, W. E. (2001). Heading and head injuries in soccer. *Sports Medicine, 31,* 369–386.

Latest fall sports study spotlights head and player contact injuries. (2001, March 12). *The NCAA News,* pp. 6, 17.

Levin, H. S., Hamsher, K. de S., & Benton, A. L. (1975). A short form of the Test of Facial Recognition for clinical use. *Journal of Psychology, 91,* 223–228.

Lezak, M. D. (1995). *Neuropsychological assessment* (3rd ed.). New York: Oxford University Press.

Macciocchi, S. N., Barth, J. T., Alves, W., Rimel, R. W., & Jane, J. A. (1996). Neuropsychological functioning and recovery after mild head injury in collegiate athletes. *Neurosurgery, 39,* 510–514.

Mathews, W. B. (1972). Footballer's migraine. *British Medical Journal, 2,* 326–327.

Matser, J. T., Kessels, A. G., Jordan, B. D., Lezak, M., & Troost, J. (1998). Chronic traumatic brain injury in professional soccer players. *Neurology, 51,* 791–796.

Matser, E. J. T., Kessels, A. G., Lezak, M. D., Jordan, B. D., & Troost, J. (1999). Neuropsychological impairment in amateur soccer players. *Journal of the American Medical Association, 282,* 971–973.

Paniak, C., Reynolds, S., Phillips, K., Toller-Lobe, G., Melnyk, A. & Nagy, J. (2002). Patient complaints within 1 month of mild traumatic brain injury: A controlled study. *Archives of Clinical Neuropsychology, 17,* 319–334.

Powell, J. W., & Barber-Foss, K. D. (1999). Traumatic brain injury in high school athletes. *Journal of the American Medical Association, 282,* 958–963.

Putukian, M., Echemendia, R. J., & Mackin, S. (2000). The acute neuropsychological effects of heading in soccer: A pilot study. *Clinical Journal of Sport Medicine, 10,* 104–109.

Reitan, R. M. (1955). The relation of the Trail Making Test to organic brain damage. *Journal of Consulting Psychology, 19,* 393–395.

Reitan, R. M., & Wolfson, D. (1999). The two faces of mild head injury. *Archives of Clinical Neuropsychology, 14,* 191–202.

Rey, A. (1941). Psychological examination of traumatic encephalopathy. *Archives de Psychologie, 28,* 286–340.

Taylor, L. B. (1969). Localization of cerebral lesions by psychological testing. *Clinical Neurosurgery, 16,* 269–287.

Tysvaer, A. & Lochen, E. (1991). Soccer injuries to the brain: A neuropsychologic study of former soccer players. *The American Journal of Sports Medicine, 19,* 56–60.

Witol, A. D., & Webbe, F. (in press). Soccer heading frequency predicts neuropsychological deficits. *Archives of Clinical Neuropsychology.*

Zachary, R. A. (1986). *Shipley Institute of living scale, revised manual.* Los Angeles: Western Psychological Services.

Original submission May 1, 2002
Accepted August 9, 2002

Applied Neuropsychology
2003, Vol. 10, No. 1, 42–47

Computer-Based Assessment of Sports-Related Concussion

Philip Schatz

Department of Psychology, Saint Joseph's University, Philadelphia, Pennsylvania, USA

Eric A. Zillmer

Department of Athletics, Drexel University, Philadelphia, Pennsylvania, USA

Sports-related concussion has received considerable attention from neuropsychologists, athletic trainers, team coaches, physicians, families, and athletes. In this context, researchers have recently developed computer programs for the assessment of sports-related concussion. Computer-based assessment of sports-related concussion saves time, allows for team baseline testing, and can be easily incorporated into the sports medicine environment. This article reviews the advantages and limitations of computer-based assessment of sports-related concussion. Within a well-coordinated concussion management program that includes input from a neuropsychologist, computer-based assessment of sports-related concussion will soon be the most common approach for assessing concussion in athletes.

Key Words: sports-related concussion, mild traumatic brain injury, neuropsychology, computerized neuropsychological assessment

Assessment of sports-related concussion has received increased attention over the past 2 decades. Over this period, neuropsychologists, athletic trainers, and other mental health professionals have attempted to understand and document the behavioral sequelae following cerebral concussions. Within this context, neuropsychological test batteries have been routinely used to determine the effects of cerebral concussion (Zillmer & Spiers, 2001). Much effort has been dedicated to outlining the parameters of neurocognitive changes following sports-related concussions for different settings, including professional football (Collins, 2001) and professional ice hockey (Echemendia & Julian, 2001); as well as for different populations, including college athletes (Barth et al., 1989; Collins et al., 1999; Lovell & Collins, 1998).

Using traditional neuropsychological assessment techniques, single, mild concussions in healthy college-aged athletes have been shown to result in decreased neurocognitive performance, with a relatively rapid recovery curve ranging from 10 days (Barth et al., 1989) up to 1 month postconcussion (Echemendia,

Putukian, Mackin, Julian, & Shoss, 2001). Cerebral concussion in individuals with a history of previous concussion (Moser & Schatz, 2002) or learning disability (Collins et al., 1999) were found to have more enduring cognitive effects. Common to all of the aforementioned studies, cerebral concussions were observed to cause at least mild deficits in attention and concentration.

Computerized testing may play a particularly important role in the sports-concussion arena. Since the neurocognitive sequelae of concussion are often represented by relatively mild symptoms, baseline testing of athletes has been shown to be a powerful assessment tool. By comparing pre- and postconcussion neuropsychological data, the neuropsychologist can differentiate changes in neurocognitive status as a result of the concussion and evaluate the degree of symptom resolution. Given the extremely large number of athletes that may benefit from a baseline-testing paradigm, paper-and-pencil tests may be too time-consuming to allow for a wide-based, baseline-testing program, particularly in high school. To this end, computer programs with accurate timing may be best suited to identify neurocognitive deficits, track progress toward recovery, and assist in return-to-play decisions, especially when postconcussive symptoms include delayed onset of response time and increased decision-making times (i.e.,

---

Requests for reprints should be sent to Philip Schatz, Assistant Professor of Psychology, St. Joseph's University, Post Hall 222, Philadelphia, PA 19131, USA. E-mail: pschatz@sju.edu reduced information processing speed). It is the intention of this article to present current trends in computer-based assessment of sports-related concussion.

Advantages and Limitations of Computer-Based Assessment

The American Psychological Association (APA) has established guidelines for computer-based tests and interpretations (APA, 1986). In doing so, the APA recognized a number of potential benefits that can be derived from the proper use of a computer in the delivery of clinical assessment services. Such benefits to the client include an improved ability to capture and engage the interest of the client, the minimization of the client's frustration and loss of dignity when working on properly constructed and presented software-based tasks, and an experience of mastery and sense of control gained by the client within the context of learning to use the computer. Benefits to the examiner include the freedom to increasingly focus on treatment or qualitative assessment gained by the automation of data collection, precise measurement of multiple domains of performance (response latency or response time in milliseconds) not possible by the human observer, and more efficient task performance such as randomization of trials or rapid modification of stimuli.

Computerized versions of tests have been found to be psychometrically equivalent when compared to traditional versions (Campbell et al., 1999; Elwood & Griffin, 1972). In the computer-based form, however, assessment measures have features that may be either absent or less accurate than when administered through traditional pencil-and-paper-based forms. These features include timing of responses and latencies, automated analysis of response patterns, transfer of results to a database for further analysis, and the ease with which normative data can be collected in a group setting (Wilson & McMillan, 1991). Computerized or automated assessment measures are, by nature, highly sensitive to subtle changes in attention, concentration, and response latency. Precise control over the presentation of test stimuli can be established, thereby increasing the reliability of computer-based tests. With computerization, the ability to control visual and auditory stimulus characteristics and features such as color, animation, and sound can be easily incorporated into all aspects of the assessment process, including the presentation of on-screen instructions (Wilson & McMillan, 1991). Thus, on general performance test measures, the speed and accuracy of differentiating visual stimuli may be superior to examiner based testing. Many of these advantages cannot be achieved with conventional testing (Kane & Reeves, 1997; Mead & Drasgow, 1993).

From a financial perspective, computer-based assessment can show cost-benefit gains over traditional administration procedures (French & Beaumont, 1987), as well as increased security of test data and patient records through computerized storage (Barak, 1999). The time and staffing requirements needed to administer and analyze a standardized battery of neurocognitive measures to an entire team of athletes can be significant. Since computer-based measures can be easily administered to groups of athletes and are scored automatically, they provide a useful tool for the consulting practitioner, team physician, or athletic trainer.

Computer-based neuropsychological test administration is not free from criticism or limitations. Test developers have often failed to meet established testing standards of reliability and validity established by the APA. Poorly designed interfaces can contribute to test anxiety on the part of the examinee. And, reductions in the amount of face-to-face interaction between the clinician and examinee can lead to misdiagnosis (Space, 1981). Furthermore, some researchers and clinicians suggest that computer-based assessment can never be equivalent to traditional methods of psychological testing, as the mode of administration creates a markedly different experience for the examinee (Honaker, 1988). In addition, computer-interface interaction may be more taxing cognitively to the concussed athlete, who may already be experiencing difficulty with attentiveness and concentration as a result of his or her injury. Thus, factors extraneous to paper-and-pencil assessments, which are introduced during computer-based assessment, must be identified and evaluated with respect to their potentially disruptive effects (Bennett, 1999).

Timing of the synchronization between the computer's microprocessor and monitor cannot occur without a measurable amount of error or delay in timing, and it can be difficult to standardize or control this delay with any degree of consistency. As a result, inaccurate timing procedures have been found in software used to assess human performance. This potentially serious technical deficiency has been well documented (Reed, 1979; Westall, Perkey, & Chute, 1986). Researchers have since developed software solutions that provide near-millisecond accuracy (Westall, Perkey, & Chute, 1989). In fact, clinicians wishing to obtain a gross measure of reaction time or response onset latency may not even require such accuracy. However, medical research efforts employing the use of functional magnetic resonance imaging (fMRI) to observe brain-behavior relationships require synching between stimuli presentation and scan acquisition within very specific time intervals (Gur et al., 2000; Gur et al., 2001). As such, fMRI technology is currently being incorporated into psychometric validation research using postconcussion and brain imaging data (Marion et al., in press) to allow accurate timing to the millisecond.

Computer-Based Neuropsychological Assessment of Sports-Related Concussion

Recently, researchers have developed computer programs for the assessment of sports-related concussion. The focus of the subsequent research has been on the utility and validation of comprehensive neuropsychological test batteries for the assessment and tracking of cognitive deficits related to sports-related concussion. Three computerized assessment approaches to assess sports-related concussion have emerged from these efforts: CogSport, HeadMinder, and the Immediate Post Concussion Assessment and Cognitive Testing (ImPACT). Comparisons among these three measures on factors such as administration time and cost, computer requirements and available technological support, data storage, and report generation procedures are presented in Table 1.

CogSport. CogSport (CogState, 1999) is a standalone software product that measures reaction time and accuracy to evaluate simple and complex attention, working memory, short-term memory and new learning, incidental memory, adaptive problem solving, continuous performance, and spatial abilities. CogSport task stimuli take the form of playing cards, which are presented either individually or grouped, with specific response requirements. Test takers respond to tasks by pressing either the D or the K on the computer's keyboard. Administration takes approximately 15 to 20 min, and results are submitted to CogState for scoring and analysis. Optional services include customized reports, custom data for import into popular statistical packages, assistance in interpretation of results for publication or presentation, assistance in the preparation of research protocols or IRB submissions, storage and retrieval of data and results, and mirroring of stored data for increased security.

CogSport was designed to evaluate changes in cognitive function, and was originally validated on approximately 300 professional Australian football play-

Table 1. *Neuropsychological Test Measures for the Computer-Based Assessment of Concussion*

Dimension	CogSport	CRI	Impact
Administration Time	15–20 min	20–25 min	20–25 min
Subtests/Tasks	Simple/Choice/Complex RT, Monitoring, One Back, Matching, Incidental & Associate Learning	Simple RT, Cued RT, Visual Recognition, Symbol Scanning, Decoding	Word Discrimination, Visual Working Memory, Sequencing, Visual Attention Span, Symbol Matching, Choice RT
Operating System	Windows 95/98/2000/NT Macintosh OS 8.6, 9, X	Internet-based: Windows- IE 5 and 6 Macintosh- Netscape 4.7	Windows 95/98/2000/NT
Administration Costs	Free to download and test $50 per report Volume discounts available for large scale projects.	High Schools $495/campus (250 baseline, 25 post-trauma) Universities $995 per campus (500 baseline, 25 post-trauma) Prof. Teams/Hospitals $1,995 (100 baseline, 25 post-trauma)	High Schools $995.00/institution (unlimited use) Universities $1,245/institution (unlimited use) Professional/other $1,495/institution (unlimited use)
Tech Support	Unlimited online support	Free online support (up to 10 e-mails); $295 for Phone support (first year)	Unlimited online and Phone support
Report Generation	$50 per athlete per year (Discounts available for bulk testing)	No additional cost Baseline comparison reports generated automatically	No additional cost Baseline comparison reports generated automatically
Data Storage	Results stored locally on user's computer or remotely on CogState's server	Results stored remotely on HeadMinder's server	Results stored on local server

Note: CRI = Concussion Resolution Index.

ers and hundreds of healthy controls across a wide range of ages (Makdissi et al., 2001). The authors indicated good test-retest coefficients and external validation with the Trail Making and Digit Symbol Substitution Tests (Collie, Darby, & Maruff, 2001). More recently, scores of 60 healthy controls on the CogSport simple and choice reaction-time tasks were compared with performance on the Digit Symbol Substitution Test and the Trail Making Test, and resultant correlation coefficients were significantly high (A. Collie, personal communication, September 2002).

Concussion Resolution Index. HeadMinder Inc., offers online neurocognitive and neurobehavioral assessment tools in the form of the Concussion Resolution Index (CRI) and Sideline Assistant (Erlanger, Feldman, & Kutner, 1999). The CRI is Internet-based, and all subtests are administered online via an Internet browser. As a result, the program is computer platform independent. Test measures are scored online, and results are accessible only to the test administrator who is responsible for interpreting and discussing test results with that athlete. The CRI is currently used by numerous professional, semipro, club, college, and high school athletic organizations on three continents.

The CRI subtests measure reaction time and speeded decision-making, and report strong concurrent validation with the Symbol Digit Modalities Test, Wechsler Adult Intelligence Scale–Third Edition Digit Symbol and Symbol Search, Grooved Pegboard, and Trail Making Tests (Erlanger et al., in press). The CRI has been found to be sensitive in identifying postconcussive symptoms, while remaining resistant to retest effects (Erlanger et al., 2001; Erlanger et al., in press). The CRI also includes an internal symptom validity measure to screen for chance responding or significantly decreased baseline test performance. The Sideline Assistant is a personal digital assistant based software application containing a roster of all athletes and pertinent medical and contact information, as well as an electronic version of the Standardized Assessment of Concussion (McCrea, Kelly, Kluge, Ackley, & Randolph, 1997).

Immediate Post Concussion Assessment and Cognitive Testing. ImPACT (Lovell, Collins, Podell, Powell, & Maroon, 2000) is a computer-based neuropsychological test battery that measures attention, memory, processing speed, and reaction time to 1/100th of a sec. The Windows-based program also consists of a selfreport symptom questionnaire and a concussion history form. Approximately 200 high

schools, intercollegiate athletic programs, and professional teams currently use ImPACT. In college football, ImPACT is utilized by 9 of the 11 Big Ten football teams, as well as teams in the Pacific-10, Southeastern Conference, and Big XII. At the professional level, ImPACT is currently in use by teams in the National Football League, Major League Baseball, the umpires of Major League Baseball, and the National Basketball Association. In addition, the Championship Auto Racing Teams and the United States Olympic Women's Hockey Team are using ImPACT.

Initial psychometric research on the ImPACT system reveals strong reliability data and validation research is in progress (Maroon et al., 2000). To date, the test developers have collected baseline data on over 5,000 athletes and have collected concussion data on approximately 340 athletes. More detailed research outlining the basic psychometrics of ImPACT (i.e., normative, reliability, and validity data) is forthcoming in the medical literature.

Discussion

When computers were first used in the 1980s for computer-based administration of psychological measures, there was much criticism directed at this new initiative. Since then, computer administered psychological tests have become more refined. As a result, psychologists have come to appreciate the many benefits of psychological tests that incorporate computer-assisted testing and interpretation (Zillmer, 1991). It seems particularly practical to use computerized neuropsychological testing for the assessment of sports-related concussions, first-and-foremost, because of the number of athletes to be tested. It is now understood that a neuropsychological baseline assessment paradigm facilitates the detection and management of mild neurocognitive changes in athletes who have sustained a concussion. The generation of objective pre- and postconcussion data is particularly important because of the transient medical symptoms often seen in this population, as well as the ambiguity of determining the severity and symptom resolution of a concussion in the absence of objective neuropsychological data. In addition, computerized testing is easy, has inherent psychometric strengths, can minimize practice effects on serial assessments, is relatively inexpensive, provides accurate reaction time measurement, and can be administered in group settings. Because of these advantages, computerized testing programs can be more easily initiated in college and high school athletic programs that often have hundreds of participants involved in sports. Because of its objectivity, computerized testing for sports-related concussions appears to have also been well received by professional teams and professional leagues within professional football, minor league hockey, and professional soccer. The future of this approach may very well be that athletic trainers and sports medicine specialists will include neuropsychological assessment in their existing protocol for the medical management of their athletes.

Most neuropsychologists critical of computerized testing will argue that such an approach removes the neuropsychologist from the scene. There certainly is some truth to this, since a comprehensive neuropsychological evaluation is best carried out in the presence of an experienced neuropsychologist (Zillmer & Ball, 1987). If one uses the forensic setting as the golden standard, perhaps because it is the most contentious, any conscientious neuropsychologist would spend considerable time with the client to obtain a neuropsychological profile. We argue, however, that the use of a widespread computerized assessment program to assess sports-related concussions will actually increase the awareness of neuropsychological services and, as a result, referrals to the neuropsychologist. Computerized assessment in sports-related concussions are very much like sophisticated screening tests; they may not provide a comprehensive evaluation of abilities, but they do provide objective evidence of neurocognitive strengths and weakness, and a pre-post comparison.

In addition, computerized tests facilitate the creation of data banks as a means of studying concussions and thus may very well prove to be a terrific vehicle for the assessment and management of this complex injury. The biggest challenge to the computerized testing approach will be on the psychometric issue of validity: "Do these tests really measure what they purport to measure?" Thus, test validity should be the most important consideration at all stages of computerized test development and test evaluation. Needless to say that a test is only as good as is its standardization. In addition, computerized tests are, of course, canned and therefore do not allow for a flexible approach to neuropsychological testing. Comprehensive neuropsychological testing may be appropriate when concussion-based symptoms do not resolve or additional emotional features arise from the injury and compromise the athlete's neurocognitive status. Finally, a standard, serial, postconcussion assessment schedule has yet to have been agreed on by researchers. The computerized testing approach would benefit from an agreed-on test retest schedule. Re-searchers and test authors are encouraged to examine this important variable.

The goal of this article was to introduce the practicing neuropsychologist to the culture of computerized neuropsychological testing, specifically as it applies to the assessment of sports-related concussions. We believe that the advantages of such an approach far outweigh its limitations. The future of sports-related concussion assessment should and will include the use of computerized baseline assessment of athletes. We introduced the three main programs that are currently on the market, although it was not our goal to provide a specific critique of each assessment approach. Documenting the reliability and validity of assessment measures may represent the most critical issue for the long-term success of computer-based assessment of sports-related concussion, in addition to establishing their utility and sensitivity to the sequelae of concussion.

References

American Psychological Association. (1986). *Guidelines for computer-based tests and interpretations.* Washington, DC: Author.

Barak, A. (1999). Psychological applications on the Internet: A discipline on the threshold of a new millennium. *Applied and Preventative Psychology, 8,* 231–245.

Barth, J. T., Alves, W. M., Ryan, T. V., Macciocchi, S. N., Rimel, R. W., Jane, J. A., et al. (1989). Head Injury in sports: Neuropsychological sequelae and recovery of function. In H. S. Levin, H. M. Eisenberg, & A. L. Benton (Eds.), *Mild head injury* (pp. 257–275). New York: Oxford University Press.

Bennett, R. E. (1999, Fall). Using new technology to improve assessments. *Educational Measurement: Issues and Practice, 18*(3), 5–12.

Brooks, J. (1998). *Epidemiology and Prevention in Youth Sports.* Lincoln: Brain Injury Association of Nebraska.

Campbell, K. A., Rohlman, D. S., Storzbach, D., Binder, L. M., Anger, W. K., Kovera, C. A., et al. (1999). Test-retest reliability of psychological and neurobehavioral tests self-administered by computer. *Assessment, 6,* 21–32.

CogState. (1999). *CogSport* [Computer software]. Parkville, Victoria, Australia: CogState, Ltd.

Collie, A., Darby, D., & Maruff, P. (2001). Computerized cognitive assessment of athletes with sports related head injury. *British Journal of Sports Medicine, 35,* 297–302.

Collins, M. (2001, November). *New developments in the management of sports-related concussions.* Paper presented at the 21st annual conference of the National Academy of Neuropsychology, San Francisco.

Collins, M. W., Grindel, S. H., Lovell, M. R., Dede, D. E., Moser, D. J., Phalin, B. R., et al. (1999). Relationship between concussion and neuropsychological performance in college football players. *Journal of the American Medical Association, 282,* 964–70.

Collins, M. W., Lovell, M. R., & Mckeag, D. B. (1999). Current issues in managing sports-related concussion. *Journal of the American Medical Association, 282,* 2283–2285.

Echemendia, R. J. (2001, November). *Return to play following sports concussion: The role of the neuropsychologist.* Paper presented at the 21st annual conference of the National Academy of Neuropsychology, San Francisco, CA.

Echemendia, R. J., & Julian, L. J. (2001). Mild traumatic brain injury in sports: Neuropsychology's contribution to a developing field. *Neuropsychology Review, 11*(2), 69–88.

Echemendia, R. J., Putukian, M., Mackin, R. S., Julian, L., & Shoss, N. (2001). Neuropsychological test performance prior to and following sports-related mild traumatic brain injury. *Clinical Journal of Sport Medicine, 11*(1), 23–31.

Elwood, D. L., & Griffin, R. (1972). Individual intelligence testing without the examiner. *Journal of Consulting and Clinical Psychology, 38*(1), 9–14.

Erlanger, D. M., Feldman, D. J., & Kutner, K. (1999). *Concussion resolution index.* New York: HeadMinder, Inc.

Erlanger, D. M., Feldman, D., Kutner, K., Kaushik, T., Kroger, H., Festa, J., et al. (in press). Development and validation of a web-based neuropsychological test protocol for sports-related return-to-play decision making. *Archives of Clinical Neuropsychology.*

Erlanger, D. M, Saliba, E., Barth, J., Almquist, J., Webright, W., & Freeman, J. (2001). Monitoring resolution of postconcussion symptoms in athletes: Preliminary results of a web-based neuropsychological protocol. *Journal of Athletic Training, 36,* 280–287.

French, C. C., & Beaumont, J. G. (1987). The reaction of psychiatric patients to computerized assessment. *British Journal of Clinical Psychology, 26,* 267–277.

Gur, R. C., Alsop, D., Glahn, D., Petty, R., Swanson, C. L., Maldjian, J. A., et al. (2000). An fMRI study of sex differences in regional activation to a verbal and a spatial task. *Brain and Language, 74,* 157–70.

Gur, R. C., Ragland, J. D., Moberg, P. J., Turner, T. H., Bilker, W. B., Kohler, C., et al. (2001). Computerized neurocognitive scanning: I. Methodology and validation in healthy people. *Neuropsychopharmacology, 25,* 766–776.

Honaker, L. (1988). The equivalency of computerized and conventional MMPI administration: a critical review. *Clinical Psychology Review, 8,* 561–577.

Kane, R. L., & Reeves, D. L. (1997). Computerized test batteries. In A. M. Horton Jr., D. Wedding, & J. Webster (Eds.), *The neuropsychology handbook: Vol. 1. Foundations and assessment* (2nd ed., pp. 423–467). New York: Springer.

Lovell, M. R., & Collins, M. W. (1998). Neuropsychological assessment of the college football player. *Journal of Head Trauma Rehabilitation, 13*(2), 9–26.

Lovell, M. R., Collins, M. W., Podell, K., Powell, J., & Maroon, J. (2000). *ImPACT: Immediate post-concussion assessment and cognitive testing.* Pittsburgh, PA: NeuroHealth Systems, LLC.

Makdissi, M., Collie, A., Maruff, P., Darby, D. G., Bush, A., McCrory, P., et al. (2001). Computerized cognitive assessment of concussed Australian Rules footballers. *British Journal of Sports Medicine, 35,* 354–60.

Marion, D.W., Lovell, M.R., Collins, M.W., Boada, F., Stenger, V.A., Field, M., et al. (in press). *fMRI and sports-related concussion.* National Institutes of Health, National Institute of Child Health and Human Development (Grant No. R01 HD42386).

Maroon, J. C., Lovell, M. R., Norwig, J., Podell, K., Powell, J. W., & Hartl, R. (2000). Cerebral concussion in athletes: evaluation and neuropsychological testing. *Neurosurgery, 47,* 659–669.

McCrea, M., Kelly, J. P., Kluge, J., Ackley, B., & Randolph, C. (1997). Standardized assessment of concussion in football players. *Neurology, 48,* 586–588.

Mead, A. D., & Drasgow, F. (1993). Equivalence of computerized and paper-and-pencil cognitive ability tests: A meta-analysis. *Psychological Bulletin, 114,* 449–458.

Moser, R. S., & Schatz, P. (2002). Enduring effects of concussion in youth athletes. *Archives of Clinical Neuropsychology, 17*(1), 81–90.

Reed, A. V. (1979). Microcomputer display timing: Problems and solutions. *Behavior Research Methods Instruments and Computers, 11,* 572–576.

Space, L. G. (1981). The computer as psychometrician. *Behavior Research Methods & Instrumentation, 13,* 595–606.

Westall, R., Perkey, M. N., & Chute, D. L. (1986). Accurate millisecond timing on Apple's Macintosh using Drexel's Millitimer. *Behavior Research Methods Instruments and Computers, 18,* 307–311.

Westall, R., Perkey, M. N., & Chute, D. L. (1989). Millisecond timing on Apple's Macintosh Revisited. *Behavior Research Methods Instruments and Computers., 21,* 540–547.

Wilson, S. L., & McMillan, T. M. (1991). Microcomputers in psychometric and neuropsychological assessment. In A. Ager (Ed.), *Microcomputers and clinical psychology: Issues, applications and future developments.* (pp. 79–94). Chichester, England: Wiley.

Zillmer, E. A. (1991). Review of the Rorschach interpretation assistance program—Version 2 computer program. *Journal of Personality Assessment, 57,* 381–383.

Zillmer, E. A., & Ball, J. D. (1987). Psychological and neuropsychological assessment in the medical setting. *Medical Times: The Journal of Family Medicine, 115,* 107–113.

Zillmer, E. A., & Spiers, M. V. (2001). *Principles of clinical neuropsychology.* Belmont, CA: Wadsworth.

Original submission May 1, 2002
Accepted August 9, 2002

Applied Neuropsychology
2003, Vol. 10, No. 1, 48–55

Return to Play Following Sports-Related Mild Traumatic Brain Injury: The Role for Neuropsychology

Ruben J. Echemendia

Department of Psychology, The Pennsylvania State University, University Park, Pennsylvania, USA

Robert C. Cantu

Division of Neurosurgery, Emerson Hospital, Concord, Massachusetts, USA

Cerebral concussions frequently occur at all levels of athletic competition. The effects from these concussions can be transient or may lead to chronic, debilitating symptoms. A growing literature has established that neuropsychological tests are useful in detecting the subtle neurocognitive changes that occur following concussions. The identification of these deficits and subsequent recovery of function can be important components in making return-to-play (RTP) decisions. This article describes the emergence of neuropsychology in sports medicine, discusses the context in which RTP decisions are made, outlines factors that are important to RTP decisions, and presents a model that views the RTP decision as a dynamic risk-benefit analysis that involves complex interactions among variables. It is argued that neuropsychology has a unique, but not exclusive, role in the decision making process. Implications for future research are discussed.

Key Words: cerebral concussions, return to play, risk-benefit analysis, neuropsychology

Interest in the area of sports neuropsychology has grown significantly over the past decade. An important reason for this interest has been the development of programs specifically geared toward the neuropsychological assessment of sport-related mild traumatic brain injury (MTBI), also known as cerebral concussion. Epidemiological data provide compelling evidence that cerebral concussions are common within contact sports at all levels of play (Powell & Barber-Foss, 1999). It has also become apparent that sports often thought to be noncontact (e.g., basketball) have athletes who sustain concussions at a relatively high rate (Putukian & Echemendia, 1996). Although concussions have traditionally been thought of as mild "dings" to the head with no discernable sequelae, we now know that the symptoms of concussion can range from highly transient annoyances to debilitating postconcussion syndrome or even death.

The combination of high prevalence rates and possible severity of the injury has captured the attention of sports medicine personnel, coaches, players, and the media. With this attention has arrived an interest in the reliable and valid assessment of MTBI. For example, the National Institute of Medicine, part of the National Academies of Science, recently sponsored a conference that examined the issue of heading in soccer players (Institute of Medicine, 2002). The primary focus of the conference was to examine neuropsychological evidence regarding repeated purposeful heading of the soccer ball. Although the panel concluded that there was no convincing evidence to date that heading leads to long-term neurocognitive dysfunction, they did call attention to the fact that concussions occur at a relatively high rate in soccer because of head-to-head, head-to-foot, and head-to-equipment (e.g., goal posts) contact.

Neuropsychology has been thrust into a unique role in the assessment of sports-related concussion. The pathophysiology of MTBI is such that it is largely invisible to traditional radiologic techniques (e.g., computed tomography, magnetic resonance imaging). Without the ability to detect the injury objectively, sports medicine physicians were forced to evaluate the injury through clinical means that were thought to be the best practices in the field. A large number of severity rating (grading) scales were developed that relied

Requests for reprints should be sent to Ruben J. Echemedia, 119 S. Burrowes St., Suite 602, State College, PA 16801, USA. E-mail: RJE2@psu.edu entirely on symptom report by athletes or direct observation by on-site personnel. There is no consensus in the field as to which grading scale should be used. These grading scales (e.g. Cantu, 1998; Colorado Medical Society, 1991; Quality Standards Subcommittee, American Academy of Neurology, 1997) divide severity into three grades that correspond to mild (I), moderate (II), and severe (III) concussions. Sets of guidelines for return-to-play (RTP) decisions were developed and correspond to each of these grades. For example, a player who sustains a Grade II concussion (no loss of consciousness, posttraumatic amnesia) under the Colorado Medical Society's grading system would be allowed to RTP after he or she was asymptomatic at rest and after exertion for 1 week. Although these grading systems and guidelines raise the awareness that cerebral concussions must be treated with caution and provide some uniformity to the management of concussion, they are not based on empirical evidence. Further, they rely solely on the self-report of athletes who are oftentimes motivated to underreport their symptoms so that they can return to competition prematurely. This is worrisome in light of Echemendia, Putukian, Mackin, Julian, and Shoss's (2001) findings that athletes' report of symptoms did not differentiate between concussed athletes and noninjured controls 48 hr following concussion, despite very significant differences in neurocognitive functioning between the two groups.

Taken together, these factors help set the stage for neuropsychology's emergence in sports medicine. Neuropsychological tests and approaches have long been used to assess neurocognitive changes following MTBI. At the University of Virginia, Barth et al. (1989) first introduced neuropsychology to sports. They were the first to use the now common paradigm of testing players at baseline and then testing the players serially postinjury. Barth et al.'s original data demonstrated that neuropsychological tests were able to detect neurocognitive changes following concussion and that these changes generally returned to baseline within 10 days of injury. These findings have been replicated across many studies, but it is beyond the scope of this article to review them. The interested reader is referred to Echemendia and Julian (2001) and Erlanger, Kutner, Barth, and Barnes (1999).

The RTP Decision

The RTP decision process is unique in neuropsychological practice because it requires that the neuropsychologist identify the point at which an injured athlete has recovered from the effects of a concussion and is able to return to a situation in which additional injury may occur. Preventing athletes from returning to sport for unnecessarily long periods of time may have significant impact on the athlete's career, financial viability, and psychological functioning. However, the importance of the RTP decision rests on the possible ramifications of a premature decision. Animal and human data have made it clear that a variety of neurochemical and structural changes occur in the brain following concussion. These data suggest that a neurochemical cascade begins within minutes of concussion and often lasts several days following concussion. During this period, neurons that have not been destroyed remain alive but in a vulnerable state. These cells are uniquely susceptible to minor changes in cerebral blood flow, increases in intracranial pressure, and, especially, anoxia. Animal studies have shown that during this period of vulnerability, a minor reduction in cerebral blood flow that would normally be inconsequential now produces extensive neuronal cell loss (Jenkins et al., 1989; Lee, Lifshitz, Hovda, & Becker, 1955; Lifshitz et al., 1955; Sutton, Hovda, Adelson, Benzel, & Becker, 1994).

The neurochemical and structural cascade has parallels in neurocognitive functioning. Several studies have documented that neurocognitive changes can exist up to 10 days following concussion (Barth et al., 1983; Collins et al., 1999). Echemendia et al. (2001) found that neuropsychological test scores, particularly with respect to verbal learning and memory, begin a process of decline that begins as early as 2 hr postconcussion and maximizes at 48 hr postinjury. Some deficits were found to exist up to 1 week following injury, but controls and concussed athletes were indistinguishable from each other at 1 month following concussion.

In light of the vulnerabilities noted previously and the possible catastrophic effects of second impact syndrome (Cantu & Voy, 1995; Kelly et al., 1991; Saunders & Harbaugh, 1984), it is clear that the RTP decision must reliably determine when the effects of the concussion have ended and the player is safe to resume competition. This is the key role for neuropsychology in sports medicine. Although useful in detecting the severity of concussion, current neuropsychological tests are not very practical in the diagnosis of concussion in sports. Diagnosis can be accomplished efficiently through sideline examinations conducted by well-trained medical personnel. Neuropsychological tests prove their usefulness in detecting the neurocognitive effects of the concussion and, more importantly, when those neurocognitive changes have returned to baseline.

The RTP Decision in Context

The RTP decision is complex and dynamic and involves many factors. It also occurs within a context that is unfamiliar to neuropsychologists. In this article, we describe the context in which the RTP is made and then elaborate a RTP model developed by Echemendia and Cantu (in press). Any neuropsychologist interested in working in this area needs to develop a good working understanding of this complex arena.

Sports teams exist within a culture in which there are multiple competing demands and a variety of interested parties that often have competing agendas. Many individuals may have impact on the RTP decision. At the professional level, there are the players, the management, coaching staff, agents, attorneys, media, family, friends, advertising contracts, and medical staff, among others. College players contend with the players on their team, the team hierarchy, the college hierarchy, medical staff, professors, their parents, girlfriends and boyfriends, scouts for professional teams, potential agents, and attorneys. At the high school level, coaches, teammates, parents, girlfriends and boyfriends, teachers, and college scouts may influence players. These individuals and their various viewpoints also interact with the level of play. As the level of play becomes more elite, the pressures intensify across all fronts. It is important to recognize the complexity of the context in which players operate because many of these individuals can potentially influence the RTP decision. Although it may be argued that RTP decisions should only involve medical factors, this perspective is likely unrealistic. In our view the RTP decision is a complex interaction of many factors with the decision maker constantly involved in a risk-benefit evaluation. It is also important to underscore that sports are competitive and frequently emotional, and decisions, including RTP decisions, are not solely based on deductive reasoning or logic.

The team physician generally holds the ultimate responsibility for the RTP decision. It is their responsibility to gather all of the necessary information and use that information to make the RTP decision. There is marked variability among physicians with respect to their involvement with the team, awareness of sports medicine, and knowledge of sport-related concussion. Some team physicians (e.g., those with professional teams and elite college teams) know the players well, travel with the teams, and are often specialty trained in sports medicine or orthopedics. At the other end of the spectrum are high school teams that rely on each player's family physician or an emergency room physi-cian to make the RTP decision. There is marked variability among these physicians regarding their experience with sports-related concussion.

Athletic trainers have often been described as the eyes and ears of the team physician. They are the members of the medical staff that work most closely with the players. They are an invaluable source of information regarding the players and the nature of their injuries. The athletic trainer is usually the first on the scene to evaluate a player, and they generally have a thorough understanding of sports-related concussion. Unfortunately, not all teams have access to athletic trainers. In high schools there may be only one full-time athletic trainer for all of the sports teams. College teams often do not travel with athletic trainers and when they do it is often the case that student trainers do the traveling. Athletic trainers are often quite busy before, during, and after athletic competition. Given their workload, it is easy for them to miss the sometimes subtle symptoms of concussion unless the player directly reports symptoms.

All teams have coaches and coaches are critical components in the management of concussion and RTP. Coaches vary in their relationships with medical staff. Some coaches view the medical staff as an integral part of the team, whereas others view the medical staff as a necessary evil. The coach sets the tone for a team both on and off the field. This is particularly true for the issue of sports concussion. If the coach recognizes the importance of careful management of concussions, the players will also appreciate the importance of the injury and more accurately report their symptoms. If, on the other hand, a coach does not believe in concussions, then detection and management of concussions becomes a very difficult process because players are encouraged to play through their symptoms and not report symptoms to medical staff. It is also important to recognize that in most youth sports the coach is the person on the field who is evaluating the severity of injuries. Since many coaches have minimal or no understanding of concussions it is likely that many children are receiving concussions and are not being evaluated or treated.

The team may also be a major influence on the RTP decision. For example, if a high-profile player is sidelined because of a concussion, the team may be tempted to pressure the medical staff into premature RTP, particularly if there is a big game at stake. A game of little or no consequence may elicit a very different response from the team. Teammates are also important factors in the identification and management of concussion. If players are educated to the signs and symptoms of concussion and they recognize the importance of the injury, they can be very helpful in detecting players who are showing the signs and symptoms of concussion. The players can accurately report if a fellow player is acting "goofy" or they are not being themselves. They know when teammates are missing plays or otherwise behaving erratically. Teammates are also quite helpful in alerting medical staff to situations where a concussed player is minimizing symptoms in order to return to competition.

Families play an important role in the RTP decision because of the integral role that they play in the lives of athletes. The family of a high school athlete who has sustained two concussions in a season may want their child to stop playing the sport because of fear of catastrophic injury. Or, parents may become angry with medical staff if their child is held out of competition because of a concussion. Often, they provide some variant of "he's tough, he can play" or "there's nothing wrong with her . . . I had a lot of worse injuries and I continued to play."

The player is also a key figure in the RTP decision. He or she is the one most directly affected by the RTP decision. It is important to speak with the player and get his or her views on returning to sport. Usually, athletes are highly motivated to return to play and consequently may minimize their symptoms. It is important to know whether the athlete will tend to minimize or, in some cases, exaggerate their symptoms. It is also critical to discuss with the athlete if they feel ready to return to competition. It is not unusual for athletes with concussions to become frightened of returning to play. They generally will not voice this fear unless asked directly.

The Role of Neuropsychology

The neuropsychologist does not usually make the RTP decision. In most instances, the neuropsychologist is a consultant to the team physician, and neuropsychological data are an important component of the RTP decision. Neuropsychologists generally become involved with concussed athletes in one of two ways: as part of an established neuropsychological testing program, where there exists baseline testing and a protocol for postinjury testing, or as a referral from a physician for a player who has had a concussion, but the player is unknown to the neuropsychologist and no baseline data exist. In both cases, the ultimate questions remain the same. Is the player suffering any neurocognitive sequelae from the concussion, can he or she return to play? The answer to these questions

is sometimes clear-cut. For example, the player data are significantly below baseline, the player is symptomatic, and he or she does not feel right. There would be general consensus that this player should not be returned to competition. The more typical scenario involves conflicting information. For example, the player is asymptomatic at rest and on exertion, yet the neuropsychological data are below baseline. Or, the neuropsychological data are only marginally below baseline. It is beyond the scope of this article to fully evaluate these issues. Since sports neuropsychology is a young field, many important basic questions remain to be answered by empirical studies. Do players need to reach baseline levels of functioning or should they actually exceed baseline levels because of practice effects? How far above or below baseline should a player perform before being allowed to return to play? How should previous concussions be included in the decision-making process? How should qualitative, process data be evaluated?

A relatively infrequent role for neuropsychologists includes evaluating players on the sideline. In this context, neuropsychologists are available to assist the team physician or athletic trainer with the RTP decision. In some cases it will be up to the team neuropsychologist to make the RTP decision. In these situations it is important that the neuropsychologist knows the players and has specialized experience working with sports teams. A thorough sideline assessment will need to be conducted. It should include assessment of motor coordination, orientation, attention and concentration, memory, information processing speed, and so on. Systematic approaches have been developed for sideline assessments (see Lovell, Echemendia, & Burke, in press; McCrea et al., 1998).

A Dynamic Model for RTP

Thus far, we have described a brief historical perspective on neuropsychology's role in sports, the various individuals who may play a role in the RTP decision, and the role of the neuropsychologist as a consultant in the RTP decision. How do these factors come together and how are they integrated in the RTP decision? We have proposed a dynamic model that attempts to capture some of the important elements in this process. Variables of interest may have direct influences on the RTP decision (e.g., whether a player has a positive magnetic resonance imaging finding or remains symptomatic), or it may have an indirect influence (e.g., affecting an upcoming big game). These variables may be grouped into the following factors: medical factors, specific concussion factors, player factors, team factors, and extraneous factors.

Medical factors have a direct influence on the RTP decision. These factors include any positive findings on neuroimaging, any abnormalities detected on comprehensive physical and neurological examination, and any player report of symptoms at rest or during exertion. The player should not be returned to sport until each of these findings has resolved completely. In the case of neuroimaging, it is possible that a structural abnormality is unexpectedly detected that may place the player at risk for brain injury. These findings need to be carefully evaluated since RTP may not be advisable.

Concussion factors include those variables that are directly related to the concussion(s) being assessed. The severity of the injury is the first factor to be evaluated. Even though there is little agreement on the grading systems for concussion, they can be helpful in assessing the severity of the injury. The absolute numbers of symptoms that a player reports as well the intensity of those symptoms are important factors to evaluate. In general, the more symptoms that a player reports, the greater the likelihood that the concussion is more severe. The level, type, and extent of any amnesia should be evaluated. The more dense the amnesia and the longer it lasts, the more severe the concussion.

Loss of consciousness (LOC) or coma has been used as a marker of concussion severity. A significant literature exists that relates length of coma to outcome among patients with traumatic brain injuries (TBI). Following the TBI literature, most of the concussions grading systems regard any LOC as the most serious type of concussion. However, the LOC that is seen on the sports field is usually momentary and rarely lasts more than 2 min. Lovell, Iverson, Collins, McKeag, and Maroon (1999) looked at the neuropsychological test performance of patients admitted to the emergency department with MTBI and found that short duration LOC was not predictive of concussion severity. Similarly, Erlanger and Kroger (2001) found no relationship between Grade III concussion and either neuropsychological test performance or duration of postconcussion symptoms. These findings have led Cantu to revise his concussion grading system to rely more on symptom duration and posttraumatic amnesia (Echemendia & Cantu, in press).

Concussion history should be carefully evaluated for any player sustaining concussion. The absolute number of concussions, their temporal relationship and duration of symptoms are all thought to be important factors in evaluating the effects of concussion. Collins et al. (1999) found that football players with two or more concussions did worse on baseline neuropsychological testing than those with one concussion or less. This study had a limited sample size and only one measure exhibited this relationship. In contrast, Macciocchi, Barth, Alves, Littlefield, and Jane (2001) found no relationship between the number of concussions and neuropsychological test data. Although there are no consistent data within sports that support the contention that multiple concussions lead to long-term neurocognitive deficits, there exists ample clinical evidence to suggest that greater care should be exercised with players who have experienced multiple concussions.

In light of the animal findings regarding the brain's vulnerability following a concussion, the temporal sequence of concussions appears to be important. The more closely spaced the concussions, the greater caution should be exercised. Also of importance are the length of symptom duration and the nature of the blow that creates the concussion. The longer symptoms last, the more severe the concussion is thought to be. The nature of the blow is important since it has been observed clinically that some players with multiple concussions exhibit symptoms with increasingly lighter blows. Whereas a very significant and direct blow to the head may be necessary to create the initial concussion, a subsequent concussion may occur with a less powerful and often indirect blow (e.g., to the posterior thorax). These cases should be carefully examined because they may signal the need to terminate a player's career.

Neuropsychological factors provide important, direct information to be used in the RTP decision. As noted earlier, neuropsychology is a newcomer to the sports medicine team, and there are many important questions that remain unanswered. However, the weight of the data that has been assembled thus far clearly suggests that neuropsychological tests are capable of detecting neurocognitive deficits as soon as 2 hr following cerebral concussion (Echemendia & Julian, 2001). These neurocognitive deficits may or may not coincide with player reported symptoms. Given the propensity for players to minimize their symptoms to return to competition, and the likelihood that they are often unaware of the cognitive deficits that they may experience, it seems prudent to keep an athlete from athletic competition until neuropsychological data are interpreted as having returned to baseline.

Player factors are often overlooked in the RTP decision, even though the player is the most important element in the decision. It is our experience that the vast majority of medical professionals who have been involved in RTP decisions agree that evaluating a player after concussions is easier, and likely more valid, when you know the player. Knowledge of the player and his or her personality is crucial in determining whether the player is exhibiting odd behavior or personality changes. The player's personality is also important in determining the aggressiveness of their play, their tendency to minimize symptoms, their willingness to follow advice, how they will respond to the concussion, and whether the player can be trusted to report any reemergence of symptoms. If the evaluating personnel do not have firsthand knowledge of the player it is important that they seek out this information from sources close to the player.

The player should have a voice in the RTP decision. This does not necessarily mean that the player will agree with the decision. Very often he or she does not agree. But involving the player in the decision helps the player understand the factors that were evaluated in the decision and generally will lead to greater acceptance of the decision by the player.

The player's skill level, career goals, and use of proper techniques are important considerations, particularly among younger athletes. Some athletes regard sports as a hobby that they enjoy and helps structure their free time. For others, sports are a prominent component of their identity. Career aspirations may need to be evaluated even though they may have indirect influence in the decision. Since any RTP decision is an assessment of risk and benefit, a physician who has a player with borderline data may be more inclined to allow an elite athlete with professional aspirations to return to sport than an athlete who does not have career goals in sports.

Team factors may also have indirect relevance to the RTP decision. The level of play (recreational vs. competitive elite or professional), team standing, team culture, importance of the game, the player's position, and the player's standing on the depth chart may all need to be evaluated in the RTP decision. These factors primarily come into consideration in the presence of equivocal data. If a player is symptomatic—has clear neurocognitive changes on testing or positive physical examination, or neuroimaging findings—the player should not be returned to play until there is return to normal functioning. However, if RTP is unclear, it is much easier to withhold an athlete from competing in a regular game than it is to keep them out of a national championship. Because less is known about the effects of concussion on younger players, it is often advisable to take a much more cautious stance with younger players than it is with older, more highly trained athletes. Sometimes the player's position is also important. For

example, a goalie in ice hockey is much less likely to sustain a concussion when compared to a forward.

Extraneous factors may also impact the RTP decision. Some physicians or coaches may consider variables such as field condition, natural versus artificial turf, traditional versus seamless glass (hockey), opposing team characteristics and fans (among others) in making the RTP decision. Some situations or conditions may increase the likelihood of reinjury.

Figure 1 depicts the dynamic interactions among these factors. As can be seen, some variables have direct and important influences on the RTP decision. Solid, bold lines depict these relationships. The number of lines suggests the strength of influence. For example, medical factors have a very strong and direct influence on the RTP decision. Neuropsychological factors also have a direct relationship to the RTP decision yet they are not as strong as the medical factors. Some factors have relationships among themselves as well as being related to the RTP decision. Neuropsychological factors and concussion factors are related to each other and both have direct effects on RTP. Player factors and team factors are bidirectional and have indirect (dotted lines) impact on RTP. On the other hand, extraneous factors are difficult to classify and have an unknown impact on the RTP decision.

Discussion

The purpose of this article was to outline and discuss the variables that are relevant to the RTP decision following sports-related MTBI and to identify a role for neuropsychological test data in that decision process. A number of variables have been identified in the context of several factors that are believed to be important considerations in the RTP process. Each concussion is different, and each player or situation is different. We have attempted to provide a model that depicts a dynamic interplay among variables. Different sets of variables come into play for each concussion and each concussion may create a unique set of interactions. We have not created a prescriptive model that attempts to classify each variable involved in the decision making process. Our goal was to create an empirically testable model that can serve as a heuristic to personnel involved in the RTP decision.

In developing this model, we are cognizant that some may argue that the only variables that should be of importance in RTP are data that are directly related to medical or neuropsychological functioning. In other words, team factors, family factors, and player issues have no

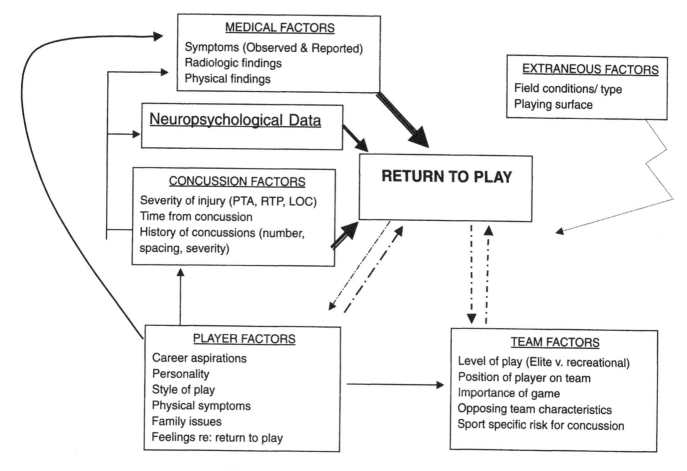

Figure 1. A dynamic model for return to play.

place in the RTP decision. Although this position may be considered by some to be an ideal, we believe that it does not reflect the struggle that is faced by physicians and other sports medicine personnel in arriving at a RTP decision. As noted at the outset, the RTP decision involves a complex risk-benefit analysis that comprises a dynamic interplay between many variables.

Neuropsychologists must be aware of the context of the RTP decision and the variables that come into play for each decision if they are to adequately serve as consultants to the team physician. Neuropsychologists have powerful clinical and research tools and an extensive knowledge base that can inform the RTP decision. Most physicians welcome and actively seek out such consultation. However, it is imperative that we keep in mind that neuropsychological factors are only one part of a complex model.

References

Barth, J. T., Macciocchi, S. N., Giordani, B., Rimel, R., Jane, J. A., & Boll, T. J. (1983). Neuropsychological sequela of minor head injury. *Neurosurgery, 13*, 529–533.

Barth, J. T., Alves, W. M., Ryan, T. V., Macciocchi, S. N., Rimel, R., Jane, J. A., et al. (1989). Mild head injury in sports: Neuropsychological sequelae and recovery of function. In H. S. Levin, H. M. Eisenberg, & A. L. Benton (Eds.). *Mild head injury* (pp. 257–275). New York: Oxford University Press.

Cantu, R. C. (1998). Return to play guidelines after head injury. *Clinical Sports Medicine, 17*, 45–60.

Cantu, R. C., & Voy, R. (1995). Second impact syndrome: A risk in any contact sport. *The Physician and Sports Medicine, 23*, 114.

Collins, M., Grindel, S., Lovell, M., Dede, D., Moser, D., Phalin, B., et al. (1999). Relationship between concussion and neuropsychological performance in college football players. *Journal of the American Medical Association, 282*, 964–970.

Colorado Medical Society. (1991). *Report of the sports medicine committee: Guidelines for the management of concussions in sports (revised)*. Denver, CO: Author.

Echemendia, R. J., & Cantu, R. (in press). Return to play following cerebral concussion. In M. Lovell, R. J. Echemendia, J. Barth, & M. Collins (Eds.), *Sports neuropsychology*.

Echemendia, R. J., & Julian, L. (2001). Mild traumatic brain injury in sports: Neuropsychology's contribution to a developing field. *Neuropsychology Review, 11*(2), 69–88.

Echemendia, R. J., Putukian, M., Mackin, R. S., Julian, L., & Shoss, N. (2001). Neuropsychological test performance prior to and following sports-related mild traumatic brain injury. *Clinical Journal of Sport Medicine, 11*, 23–31.

Erlanger, D., & Kroger, H. (2001). A clinical investigation of sports-related concussion grading scales. *Archives of Clinical Neuropsychology, 16,* 740.

Erlanger, D., Kutner, K., Barth, J., & Barnes .(1999). Neuropsychology of sports-related head injury: Dementia pugilistica to post concussion syndrome. *The Clinical Neuropsychologist, 13,* 193–209.

Jenkins, L. W., Moszynski, K., Lyeth, B. G., Lewelt, W., DeWitt, D. S., Allen, A., et al. (1989). Increased vulnerability of the mildly traumatized brain to cerebral ischemia: The use of controlled secondary ischemia as a research tool to identify common or different mechanisms contributing to mechanical and ischemic brain injury. *Brain Research, 477,* 211–224.

Institute of Medicine. (2002). *Is soccer bad for children's heads? Summary of the IOM workshop on neuropsychological consequences of head impact in youth soccer.* Washington, DC: National Academy Press.

Kelly, J. P., Nichols, J. S., Filley, C. M., Lillehei, K. O., Rubinstein, D., & Kleinschmidt-DeMasters, B. K. (1991). Concussion in sports: Guidelines for the prevention of catastrophic outcome. *Journal of the American Medical Association, 266,* 2867–2869.

Lee, S. M., Lifshitz, J., Hovda, D. A., & Becker, D. P. (1955). Focal cortical-impact injury produces immediate and persistent deficits in metabolic autoregulation [Abstract]. *Journal of Cerebral Blood Flow Metabolism, 15,* s722.

Lifshitz, J., Pinanong, P., et al. (1955). Regional uncoupling of cerebral blood flow and metabolism in degenerating cortical areas following a lateral cortical contusion [Abstract]. *Journal of Neurotrauma, 12,* 129.

Lovell, M., Echemendia, R., & Burke, K. (in press). Neuropsychological assessment in professional hockey. In M. Lovell, R. Echemendia, J. Barth, & M. Collins (Eds.), *Sports neuropsychology.* Lisse, The Netherlands: Swets & Zeitlinger.

Lovell, M., Iverson, G., Collins, M., McKeag, D., & Maroon, J. (1999). Does loss of consciousness predict neuropsychological decrements after concussion? *Clinical Journal of Sport Medicine, 9,* 193–198.

Macciocchi, S. N., Barth, J. T., Alves, W. A., Littlefield, L., & Jane, J. A. (2001). Multiple concussions and neuropsychological functioning in college football players. *Journal of Athletic Training, 36,* 303–306.

McCrea, M., Kelly, J. P., Randolf, C., Kluge, J., Bartolic, E., Finn, G., et al. (1998). Standardized assessment of concussion: On-site mental status evaluation of the athlete. *Journal of Head Trauma Rehabilitation, 13,* 27–35.

Powell, J. W., & Barber-Foss, K. D. (1999). Traumatic brain injury in high school athletes. *Journal of the American Medical Association, 282,* 958–962.

Putukian, M., & Echemendia, R. J. (1996). Managing successive minor head injuries: Which tests guide return to play? *Physician and Sportsmedicine, 24,* 25–38.

Quality Standards Subcommittee, American Academy of Neurology (1997). Practice parameter: The management of concussion in sports (summary statement). *Neurology, 48,* 581–585.

Saunders, R. L., & Harbaugh, R. E. (1984). The second impact in catastrophic contact-sports head trauma. *Journal of the American Medical Association, 252,* 538–539.

Sutton, R. L., Hovda, D. A., Adelson, P. D., Benzel, E. C., & Becker, D. P. (1994). Metabolic changes following cortical contusion: Relationships to edema and morphological changes. *Acta Neurochrurgica, 6,* 466–448.

Original submission May 1, 2002
Accepted August 9, 2002

Subscription Order Form

Please ☐ enter ☐ renew my subscription to:

Applied Neuropsychology

Volume 10, 2003, Quarterly — ISSN 0908–4282/Online ISSN 1532–4826

SUBSCRIPTION PRICES PER VOLUME:

Category:	Access Type:	Price: US/All Other Countries
☐ Individual	Online & Print	$90.00/$120.00

Subscriptions are entered on a calendar-year basis only and must be paid in advance in U.S. currency—check, credit card, or money order. Prices for subscriptions include postage and handling. Journal prices expire 12/31/03. **NOTE:** Institutions must pay institutional rates. Individual subscription orders are welcome if prepaid by credit card or personal check. **Please note:** A $20.00 penalty will be charged against customers providing checks that must be returned for payment. This assessment will be made only in instances when problems in collecting funds are directly attributable to customer error.

☐   **Check Enclosed** (U.S. Currency Only)   Total Amount Enclosed $_____

☐   **Charge My:** ☐ VISA   ☐ MasterCard   ☐ AMEX   ☐ Discover

Card Number _____   Exp. Date_____/_____

Signature_____

(Credit card orders cannot be processed without your signature.)
PRINT CLEARLY for proper delivery. STREET ADDRESS/SUITE/ROOM # REQUIRED FOR DELIVERY.

Name_____

Address_____

City/State/Zip+4_____

Daytime Phone#_____E-mail address_____
Prices are subject to change without notice.

Mail orders to: Lawrence Erlbaum Associates, Inc., Journal Subscription Department
10 Industrial Avenue, Mahwah, NJ 07430; (201) 258–2200; FAX (201) 760–3735; journals@erlbaum.com

Library Recommendation Form

Detach and forward to your librarian.

☐ I have reviewed the description of *Applied Neuropsychology* and would like to recommend it for acquisition.

Applied Neuropsychology

Volume 10, 2003, Quarterly — ISSN 0908–4282/Online ISSN 1532–4826

Category:	Access Type:	Price: US/All Other Countries
☐ Institutional	Online & Print	$380.00/$410.00
☐ Institutional	Online Only	$340.00/$340.00
☐ Institutional	Print Only	$340.00/$370.00

Name_____Title_____

Institution/Department_____

Address_____

E-mail Address_____

Librarians, please send your orders directly to LEA or contact from your subscription agent.

Lawrence Erlbaum Associates, Inc., Journal Subscription Department
10 Industrial Avenue, Mahwah, NJ 07430; (201) 258–2200; FAX (201) 760–3735; journals@erlbaum.com

---

FOR INFORMATION ON *APPLIED NUEROPSYCHOLOGY* SUBSCRIPTIONS:
CALL TOLL-FREE **1-800-926-6579**
E-MAIL LEA AT **journals@erlbaum.com**
OR VISIT LEA ONLINE AT **www.erlbaum.com**

Contributor Information

MANUSCRIPT PREPARATION: Use a word processor to prepare manuscript. Using $8\frac{1}{2}$- × 11-in. nonsmear paper, type all components (a) double-spaced, (b) 1,800 to 2,000 characters per page (70 to 75 characters per line [including spaces] × 25 to 27 lines per page), (c) on one side of the paper, (d) with each component beginning on a new page, and (e) in the following order—title page (p. 1), abstract (p. 2), text (including quotations), references, appendices, footnotes, tables, and figure captions. Consecutively number all pages (including photocopies of figures). Indent all paragraphs.

Title Page and Abstract: On page 1, type (a) article title, (b) author name(s) and affiliation(s), (c) running head (abbreviated title, no more than 45 characters and spaces), (d) acknowledgments, and (e) name and address of the person to whom requests for reprints should be addressed. On page 2, type an abstract ($\leq$ 150 words) and key words ($\leq$ 8).

Editorial Style and References: Prepare manuscripts according to the *Publication Manual of the American Psychological Association* (5th ed., 2001; APA Order Department, P.O. Box 2710, Hyattsville, MD 20784 USA). Follow "Guidelines to Reduce Bias in Language" (*APA Manual*, pp. 61–76).

Double-space references. Compile references alphabetically (see *APA Manual* for multiple-author citations and references). Spell out names of journals. Provide page numbers of chapters in edited books. Text citations must correspond accurately to the references in the reference list.

Tables: Refer to *APA Manual* for format. Double-space. Provide each table with explanatory title; make title intelligible without reference to text. Provide appropriate heading for each column in table. Indicate clearly any units of measurement used in table. If table is reprinted or adapted from another source, include credit line. Consecutively number all tables.

Figures and Figure Captions: Figures should be (a) high-resolution illustrations or (b) glossy, high-contrast black-and-white photographs.

Do not clip, staple, or write on back of figures; instead, write article title, figure number, and *TOP* (of figure) on label and apply label to back of each figure. Consecutively number figures. Attach photocopies of all figures to manuscript.

Consecutively number captions with Arabic numerals corresponding to the figure numbers; make captions intelligible without reference to text; if figure is reprinted or adapted from another source, include credit line.

COVER LETTER, PERMISSIONS, CREDIT LINES: In cover letter, include contact author's postal and e-mail addresses and phone and fax numbers.

Only original manuscripts will be considered for publication in *Applied Neuropsychology*. The cover letter should include a statement that the findings reported in the manuscript have not been previously published and that the manuscript is not being simultaneously submitted elsewhere.

Authors are responsible for all statements made in their work and for obtaining permission to reprint or adapt a copyrighted table or figure or to quote at length from a copyrighted work. Authors should write to original author(s) and original publisher to request nonexclusive world rights in all languages to use the material in the article and in future editions. Include copies of all permissions and credit lines with the manuscript. (See p. 175 of *APA Manual* for sample credit lines.)

MANUSCRIPT SUBMISSION: Submit four (4) high-quality manuscript printouts to the Editor:

B. P. Uzzell
Memorial Neurological Association
7777 Southwest Freeway, Suite 900
Houston, TX 77074 USA

MANUSCRIPT REVIEW AND ACCEPTANCE: All manuscripts are peer reviewed.

Authors of accepted manuscripts submit (a) disk containing two files (word-processor and ASCII versions of final version of manuscript), (b) printout of final version of manuscript, (c) camera-ready figures, (d) copies of all permissions obtained to reprint or adapt material from other sources, and (e) copyright-transfer agreement signed by all co-authors. Use a newly formatted disk and clearly label it with journal title, author name(s), article title, file names (and descriptions of content), names of originating machine (e.g., IBM, Mac), and word processor used.

It is the responsibility of the contact author to ascertain that all co-authors approve the accepted manuscript and concur with its publication in the journal.

Content of files must exactly match that of manuscript printout, or there will be a delay in publication. Manuscripts and disk are not returned.

PRODUCTION NOTES: Authors' files are copyedited and typeset into page proofs. Authors read proofs to correct errors and answer editors' queries.

For Product Safety Concerns and Information please contact our EU
representative GPSR@taylorandfrancis.com Taylor & Francis Verlag GmbH,
Kaufingerstraße 24, 80331 München, Germany

Printed and bound by CPI Group (UK) Ltd, Croydon, CR0 4YY
01/05/2025
01858593-0001